health

AND

human

flourishing

RELIGION,

MEDICINE,

AND

MORAL

ANTHROPOLOGY

CAROL TAYLOR, C.S.F.N.

and ROBERTO DELL'ORO, *Editors*

GEORGETOWN UNIVERSITY PRESS | WASHINGTON, D.C.

As of January 1, 2007, 13-digit ISBN numbers will replace
the current 10-digit system.
Paperback: 978-1-58901-079-6
Cloth: 978-1-58901-078-9

Georgetown University Press, Washington, D.C.

LIBRARY OF CONGRESS CATALOGING-IN-PUBLICATION DATA
Health and human flourishing : religion, medicine, and
moral anthropology
    / Carol Taylor, and Roberto dell'Oro, editors.
    p.   cm.
    Includes bibliographical references and index.
    ISBN-13: 978-1-58901-078-9 (cloth : alk. paper)
    ISBN-10: 1-58901-078-7 (cloth : alk. paper)
    ISBN-13: 978-1-58901-079-6 (pbk. : alk. paper)
    ISBN-10: 1-58901-079-5 (pbk. : alk. paper)
    1. Health—Religious aspects—Catholic Church.
2. Theological anthropology. 3. Bioethics—Religious
aspects—Catholic Church. 4. Medical ethics—Religious
aspects—Catholic Church. 5. Christian ethics—Catholic
authors. 6. Catholic Church—Doctrines. I. Taylor, Carol,
CSFN. II. Dell'Oro, Roberto, 1959–   .
    [DNLM: 1. Bioethics. 2. Anthropology, Cultural.
3. Catholicism. 4. Ethics, Medical.   WB 60 H4335 2006]
    BX1795.H4H96 2006
      261.8'321—dc22

                                    2005027251

This book is printed on acid-free paper meeting the
requirements of the American National Standard for
Permanence in Paper for Printed Library Materials.

13 12 11 10 09 08 07 06   9 8 7 6 5 4 3 2
First printing

Printed in the United States of America

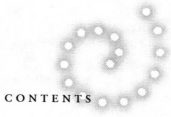

CONTENTS

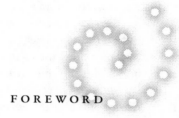

FOREWORD

The Center for Clinical Bioethics at Georgetown University is a university-based ethics resource for those who shape and give health care. Its mission reads:

> Committed to the dynamic interplay between theory and practice, experience and reflection, Center scholars bring expertise in theology, philosophy, basic science and clinical practice to today's ethical challenges. We seek to promote serious ethical reflection and discourse in pursuit of a just society and health care that affirms the dignity and social nature of all persons.

This volume is the outcome of just such serious, and interdisciplinary, ethical reflection and discourse. As our faculty grappled with how best to think about the "promises and perils" of new medical discoveries, emerging biotechnologies, and unprecedented social change, we repeatedly bemoaned the absence of a rich theological anthropology for bioethics. Drawing on our respective disciplines, we devoted numerous works-in-progress to efforts identifying what theology, philosophy, science, and medicine claim about what it means to be human and to an exploration of whether or not these beliefs ought to hold normative value.

In the earliest days of this project, urged by Warren Lux and Roberto Dell'Oro, we focused specifically on the fact of human vulnerability. We tried to envision how American bioethics would have evolved had responsiveness to vulnerability been one of the Beauchamp and Childress core principles, standing proudly with beneficence, nonmaleficence, autonomy, and justice. It became apparent, however, that what we really wanted to do was to ask more foundational questions about human health and flourishing, while standing deeply in the Roman Catholic faith tradition. We envisioned a symposium with reflective scholars who would ponder with us the *what* and *why* of a theological rather than a philosophical anthropology and what the content of such an anthropology would be. The result was a set of commissioned papers. We then met for two long and rich days of dialogue about the ideas and concepts discussed in our writings, after which we revised our papers, and those writings have evolved into the chapters of this book. It should be noted that the chief criteria for being invited to work on this project was not holding a particular set of religious convictions, but rather holding a history of scholarship evidencing careful reflection on what it means to be human and demonstrating respect for those who approach the question from a particular faith tradition. The end product is more diverse in its perspectives than we had envisioned and far richer. It aptly illustrates the fruit of the type of dialogue that characterizes the moral community at the Center.

We first want to thank the scholars who accepted our invitation to work on this project. Many of us found our two days together to be a highlight of the academic year and wished for more opportunities to devote to such exchange. We also benefited greatly from colleagues who reviewed our papers and joined us for the two days of dialogue: Robert Barnet; Richard Brown; Peter Clark, S.J.; Fr. Don Stefano Cucchetti; Alfonso Gomez-Lobo; John Collins Harvey; John Keown; Brian McDermott, S.J.; Michele Langowski; Warren Lux; Leslie Meltzer; David Miller; Kathleen Neill; Ed Neill; Kevin O'Rourke, O.P.; Warren Reich; and Jack Sisson. Brian McDermott, S.J., also offered us his support in securing the Riggs Library for our discussions, a perfect setting for the symposium. Of course, no project of this magnitude would exist without the superb efficiency of the "person behind the scenes" who was absolutely committed to making this work and who coordinated all our schedules. Thank you, Marti Patchell. To Marilee LeBon, who painstakingly edited the manuscript, ensured a better read, and got us to the publisher on schedule, our great gratitude.

INTRODUCTION

Roberto Dell'Oro

Since its birth, bioethics has been concerned with questions of meaning pertaining to health, suffering, and death, and with ethical judgment on the direction undertaken by the life sciences in their advances, especially over the last decades. This book offers a singular contribution to the interplay of religion, medicine, and moral anthropology in the field of bioethics as it struggles to articulate the conditions that define human flourishing in the age of science and technology.

This task calls for preliminary clarifications. In particular the engagement of medicine with religion and moral anthropology betrays an understanding of bioethics that pushes the boundary of current discussions, mainly focused on questions of harms, benefit, patient autonomy, and the equality of health care distribution. Although, at a normative level, those questions are inescapable and need to be squarely faced, they remain, nevertheless, within the ethical space already predefined by technological progress.

For the authors of this book, bioethics is not just a function of immanence, relative to the development of the life sciences and the place of ethical discourse within them. Because of its concern with human flourishing, bioethics also can speak with the language of "otherness," calling medical development to an ultimate understanding that necessarily presupposes *critical* distance. In this latter sense, bioethics mediates a function of transcendence, a form of mindfulness that impels medical progress toward its own telos. With Edmund Pellegrino, one might say that such a telos can only be achieved in an attitude of faithfulness to the "internal morality of medicine."[1] At the same time, because it articulates the ends of medicine in the context of a communal ethos, with its needs, values, and priorities, bioethics must be understood as a function of critical analysis that borrows from the anthropological milieux in which it operates. The internal morality of medicine articulates itself in a dynamic process, unfolding through the concrete intermediation with particular ideologies of human fulfillment.[2] This latter consideration commands an appreciation for the disclosure of meaning relative to history and for the truth of the *humanum* that inhabits the social context in which medicine operates.

This book sees bioethics as serving a twofold commitment to the *anamnesis of meaning*, one that has been hindered in the medical context by the limited vision of positivist natural sciences and, in ethics, by an excessive preoccupation with normative dimensions.[3] The former is a recurring temptation of medicine, most visible of late in the discussions on matters of genetics and research.

As for the latter, search for meaning entails a disposition to listen to rich anthropological dimensions that always inform our conception of right and wrong, good or bad. A bioethics thus conceived offers more than a purely regulatory framework, requiring periodical rearrangements on the "internal coherence" of the system being developed.[4] Indeed, openness to the latest normative integration, in an endless exercise of "reflective equilibrium," might not suffice if such a system fails to address "deepest matters of our humanity." Brilliant moral theories might come too late, when our humanity has already lost its soul.[5] A deeper analysis of our anthropological condition is needed.

Consider the meaning of such statements in relation, for example, to the question of vulnerability. Few observations appear more commonplace or seem more obvious than the observation that vulnerability is an intrinsic part of the human condition. The fluctuating differentials in power between and among individual human beings result in political, economic, social, and other forms of vulnerability. These forms of vulnerability contribute to the way in which relationships with others are defined, modifying those relations as power shifts. At one time or another, we have all been vulnerable to others, and others have been vulnerable to each of us. There are, of course, other inescapable and universal vulnerabilities. Everyone is vulnerable to accidents, illness, disability, and ultimately, death. In particular, health care professionals experience vulnerability at two different levels: the first referring to the vulnerability that exists in a relationship of differential power in which the health care professional or the investigator has a special expertise not available to the patient, or to the subject of research; and the second referring to the vulnerability related to the existential experience of impaired well-being and the associated awareness of eventual, perhaps imminent death.

All things considered, then, one would think that vulnerability has played a central role in the history of our formal thought about ethics in general and about bioethics in particular. Yet, as Alasdair McIntyre has pointed out, "the history of the Western moral philosophy suggests otherwise. From Plato to Moore and since there are, usually, with some rare exceptions, only passing references to human vulnerability and affliction and to the connections between them and our dependence on others."[6] However, in the index of what is arguably the most influential work and the most widely used approach to bioethics in America, *Principles of Biomedical Ethics,* by Beauchamp and Childress, vulnerability is not even mentioned.[7]

The reason for what could be termed the demise of vulnerability in ethics would require a long historical analysis. Suffice it to say that the lack of attention to vulnerability reflects a particular representation of the moral subject, one that stands in the effective history of post-Cartesian philosophy as well as a general idealization of the meaning of moral experience inspired by rationalistic hermeneutics of the moral event. Both Kantian and utilitarian versions of moral philosophy, though considerably different in their anthropological presuppositions, are joined by similar representations of the moral subject as autonomous, individualistic, and self-sufficient. Such a representation persists also in more recent expressions of Kantian and utilitarian moral philosophy.

The relationship between ethical principles and ideas and larger anthropological constructions of the human self has come under increased scrutiny in postmodern versions of ethical discourse, from Emanuel Levinas to

Paul Ricoeur and Jean Luc Marion, to name but a few.[8] Thus the retrieval of vulnerability in ethics could be made possible by a concentration on the historical and contextual dimensions of ethical discourse and, more broadly, on the phenomenological meaning of specific realms of human moral experience hitherto neglected. This is precisely the task that *Health and Human Flourishing* intends to fulfill as it surveys broader aspects of the human condition—from dignity and integrity to vulnerability and relationality—that are relevant to bioethical discourse.

The book is divided into six sections. In part 1, "Questioning at the Boundary," preliminary methodological issues are being addressed. Looking at the relation between theological anthropology and bioethics, Roberto Dell'Oro, in chapter 1, claims that in the Christian tradition both the *form* and the *content* of theological anthropology remain constantly open to the task of new philosophical reinterpretations. At the same time, although one might encounter within moral theology different interpretive models of the relation between faith and moral reason, it remains undisputable that faith in the Christian revelation generates a particular anthropological preunderstanding. Faith elicits reflection from moral reason and inspires moral reason. In doing so, it produces a *specific* horizon of meaning, or a "system of anthropological coordinates" from which the believer sees himself/herself and the world.

Approaching the anthropological question from a phenomenological point of view, in chapter 2, Alisa Carse points to the prevailing ethical discourse as illustrated by moral models of responsible agency that emphasize our capacity for self-control, self-determination, and independence. Yet a thoughtful look at the human predicament renders the concept of the "in-control agent" more of a fantasy than a useful moral paradigm. Vulnerability to disability, loss, and suffering are inescapable dimensions of the human condition, making it difficult—even, at times, impossible—for us to manage alone. Carse examines the role of vulnerability both in human affliction and in human thriving. Her chapter highlights one form of vulnerability in particular, namely our dignitary vulnerability, that is, our susceptibility to the degrading attitudes of others and to self-denigration and shame, often (ironically) provoked by our vulnerabilities themselves. It is generally acknowledged that we are, among the universe of creatures, capable of distinctive forms of self-creation and responsibility. In light of this, the challenge arises as to how, in honestly embracing our susceptibilities and dependencies, we can exercise responsibility in creating forms of connection through which we can flourish as humans. A crucial response to this challenge is found in the cultivation and exercise of the virtues of empathy, compassion, and solidarity. These constitute forms of human connection and social practice responsive to human need. Accepting vulnerability and allowing ourselves to be vulnerable is not an "indignity" but a crucial dimension of our capacity to sustain a felt sense of dignity and effective agency in the face of life's challenges and tragic turns.

In the final chapter of part 1, William Desmond explores the anthropological condition as defined by the relation to truth. He argues that there is a strong contemporary tendency to stress pluralism of truths and that human beings are *constructive* of their own truth. Yet, Desmond points out, while we do not possess absolute truth, a radical skepticism does not make sense, and there is more at issue than the pluralism of constructed truths. As creatures of the "between," we are not devoid of relation to truth; this is crucially evident in the exigence to be truthful that human beings know intimately. Indeed, there is a patience to truth that precedes our own efforts at construction. This patience is not something toward which we should take a merely negative relation, such as the will to conquer it entirely through our constructivist interventions. Whereas the active nature of human existence is not denied, there is a patience to being whose elemental nature is not to be denied either. This patience is consonant with an understanding of what it means to be human, an understanding whose consequences are explored in a diversity of directions, especially the vulnerable finitude of the human being and its manifestation in the practices of medicine.

Part 2 explores the meanings of "Dignity and Integrity." With a reflection inspired by analytic philosophy, Dan Sulmasy sets out in chapter 4 to explore the meaning of intrinsic dignity. He suggests that there are two basic types of values, attributed and intrinsic. Attributed values are conferred upon individuals, processes, or states of affairs by a valuer. One example of attributed values are the so-called instrumental values because they depend upon the purposes of the valuer. By contrast, intrinsic values are those that something has by virtue of its being the kind of thing that it is, independent of any attribution of value. Arguing that the concept of an intrinsic value presumes the concept of natural kinds, Sulmasy pleads for a form of "modest essentialism." The intrinsic value of the most valuable kind of thing we know is the value that a human being has by virtue of being the kind of thing a human being is. This, Sulmasy suggests, is what is meant by intrinsic dignity.

Shedding further light on the nature of integrity, Margaret Mohrmann, in chapter 5, claims that integrity refers to two qualities of a human being. First, integrity denotes the characteristic of being consistent with one who has been divinely created and, over time, formed to be. Here ongoing formation imparts a certain flexibility to integrity, as opposed to a rigidity of response and attitude; at the same time, the original, created form provides limits to that flexibility and grounds common usage of "integrity" as an indicator of moral goodness. Second, integrity denotes the human characteristic of being a unified whole, whose parts or aspects are inseparable and nonhierarchically integrated such that violations of one part must be understood, ceteris paribus, as violations of the whole. Mohrmann works out the significant implications of this argument for bioethics, or any ethics of medicine, in its understanding of human health and the response to illness.

Suzanne Holland, in chapter 6, looks at the question of integrity by noting that in bioethics the conversation on integrity most commonly takes place in research ethics. We are all loath to repeat the horrors of Tuskegee, and so we design research studies with what we hope is integrity—that is to say, we aim first of all to protect the dignity and vulnerability of the persons in our studies. This we do through informed consent, and through the principle of autonomy. But little of this, while laudable, is helpful in the many cases that come to us outside of the research arena. Holland shows the meaning of integrity by analyzing, first, the theological context in which the category emerges. Her analysis focuses on whether integrity tells us anything at all about being a human before God. Is it a helpful concept as we sort through the practical muddles of bioethics? After examining the origins and context of integrity she considers the case of elective cosmetic surgery, specifically breast augmentation, offering a framework for corporeal integrity that attempts to integrate a theological ethics into a realm that has largely been the province of philosophical bioethics.

Three chapters in part 3 deal with "Vulnerability." In chapter 7, S. Kay Toombs explores the experience of vulnerability and the meaning of illness through a reflection on her experience as a person living with multiple sclerosis. In the first part of her chapter, Toombs discusses three primary manifestations of vulnerability in illness: the perception of the body threat, the transformation of the familial world, and the threat to personal integrity, noting how cultural attitudes regarding all such things as health, independence, physical appearance, and mortality accentuate the lived experience of vulnerability and increase the patient's suffering. Furthermore, such cultural attitudes reflect an impoverished view of human flourishing. In the second part of the chapter, Toombs suggests that authentic Christian communities may offer an alternative culture with a significantly different value system—one that changes the meaning of vulnerability in illness and enhances personal integrity.

Following in the same phenomenological mode, Richard Zaner, in chapter 8, highlights the central context within which vulnerability is situated: the clinical encounter between helpers and those who appeal for help. This relationship is fundamentally asymmetrical, with power on the side of the provider in contrast to the vulnerability of the patient. The mythic sources of the fundamental moral enigma—why not take advantage of the vulnerable person?—present this theme dramatically: Plato's portrayal of the Gyges legend against the Hippocratic tradition. Illness is a key way in which an otherwise dormant moral sense can be awakened and carried out clinically by means of concrete conversation and plain talk. Because every clinical encounter is essentially haunted by the temptation to take advantage of the vulnerable, it is also challenged by the invitation to be responsive.

In the final chapter of part 3, chapter 9, Therese Lysaught argues that the philosophical anthropology that dominates medicine and bioethics too often reduces human identity to rationality and autonomy, individualistically construed. Yet for such an anthropology, the realities of illness—a sine qua non of medicine and bioethics—stand as anomalies. Illness quickly marshals empirical evidence against its truth claims. Rather than standing as a confounding glitch, illness and healing have been central to the Christian tradition since its beginning. What one finds in early Christian sources is easy to miss or dismiss, given our habit of reading such narratives and practices with lenses shaped by modern philosophy. But if we listen carefully to these sources, we will, Lysaught submits, discover a more accurate and adequate account of who we are and what it means for us to flourish. This chapter establishes a first step in developing a more truthful anthropology for bioethics, namely, a *theological* anthropology.

Part 4, "Relationality," examines dimensions of sexual and social anthropology. In chapter 10, Christine Gudorf reviews new scientific and social scientific discoveries that have challenged the reigning paradigm of human sexual anthropology without providing any successor candidate. Discoveries that neither gender roles nor sexual orientation are determined by biological sex have been followed by challenges to sexual dimorphism. Sex, as well as sexual orientation, seems to exist on a spectrum, depending on which biological marker of sexuality is chosen. Thus, all prevailing

norms in which maleness or femaleness or sexual orientation are involved
are also questionable, insofar as they assume that we know to what extent
any of these biological markers determine behavior. Gudorf concludes with
applications to the field of bioethics.

Writing from the perspective of the Christian social tradition, Lisa
Sowle Cahill, in chapter 11, maintains that the Christian view of human
relationality is built on the basic human experience of interdependence
with others in community. Human interdependence provides common
ground for talking about the good society, and about defining the meaning of justice for bioethics. Although human societies are always marked
by competition and conflict, there is an equally universal human need for
and drive toward cooperation. Religious narratives can be powerful agents
in motivating and shaping cooperation. The Christian tradition does so
with doctrines and symbols such as Creation, the image of God, universal
salvation in Christ, and "the preferential option for the poor" based on
Jesus' ministry. Moreover, the Catholic common good tradition emphasizes sociality, participation, and solidarity, as well as empowerment of the
poor. A Christian anthropology of relationships and interdependence in
the common good must be carried beyond general principles and values to
concrete practices. The author concludes with some practical illustrations
from health care, focusing on the Catholic Health Association and global
AIDS activism under Catholic auspices.

Part 5 analyzes the relation between theological anthropology and
the realms of health care, policy, and science. In chapter 12, Carol Taylor
addressed the first sphere, claiming that a rich theological anthropology
would provide guidance on, at the least, the following: how to find meaning in the vulnerabilities that accompany birth, aging and its developmental challenges, acute and chronic illness and dying; organize and deliver
health care; how to approach all parties receiving and providing health
care, especially the most vulnerable; how to make individual health care
decisions as both patients/surrogates and health care professionals; and,
finally, how to prioritize health decisions as institutions.

Ron Hamel, in chapter 13, then looks at the potential contributions
of a theological anthropology to health policy. His essay examines three
questions: (1) Why does health policy need a theological anthropology?
(2) What might a theological anthropology contribute to public policy,
generally and specifically? (3) What are some of the challenges that a theological anthropology faces in relation to health policy? Despite a number
of significant challenges, a theological anthropology has the potential to
make important contributions to the shaping of health policy. In brief, it

helps expand our moral imaginations so that we will not one day regret the policy choices we make today. These will be choices that truly respect human dignity and contribute to human flourishing.

Chapter 14, by Kevin FitzGerald, looks at the difficult question of how theological anthropology might engage in active reflection upon and interaction with the findings of the natural sciences. FitzGerald moves from the realization that our understanding of human anatomy and physiology, human development, biochemistry, genetics, and psychology—in short, every aspect of human nature that has been examined and investigated by the natural sciences—has changed radically over the course of history, particularly over the past several decades. Because of such radical shifts of paradigms, scientific investigation and biotechnological innovation are bound to bring with them new challenges to our conceptions of human nature, human flourishing, and theological anthropology.

Edmund D. Pellegrino concludes the book by surveying the varying anthropologies for the field of bioethics. His reflections are grounded on the assumption that philosophical anthropology is the foundation stone on which the theory and content of any system of bioethics is ultimately set. Although the question "what is man?" can no longer be taken for granted, it is, in the end, our answer to it that frames the wide range of different norms, principles, values, or intuitions that characterize today's bioethical discourse. If we do not know who and what it means to be human, how can we judge whether the prodigious powers of biomedical science threaten or enhance our humanity? Where else can we find the template with which to measure our attempts to benefit humankind?

All these questions might be better left open for the readers themselves to ponder. This book serves as a stimulus to think further rather than as a storehouse of ready-made answers. Through a variety of philosophical methodologies, comprising analytical, phenomenological, hermeneutical, and historical approaches, and open to the ultimate thrust of human mindfulness, where the "secular" borders on the "religious," the book offers itself as a simple, unpretentious *donne à penser*. The editors and contributors hope that it will lead to a richer bioethics.

NOTES

1. See Edmund Pellegrino, "The Internal Morality of Clinical Medicine: A Paradigm for the Ethics of the Helping and Healing Profession," *The Journal of Medicine and Philosophy* 26 (2001): 559–79. The entire issue of that journal is dedicated to a discussion of Pellegrino's "internal morality of medicine" with

contributions by Robert Veatch, Tom Beauchamp, Franklin Miller, Howard Brody, and John Arras.

2. For the debate on the goals of medicine, see Mark J. Hanson and Daniel Callahan, *The Goals of Medicine: The Forgotten Issue in Health Care Reform* (Washington, DC: Georgetown University Press, 1999).

3. For a thorough discussion of this point, see Warren Reich (with the assistance of Roberto Dell'Oro), "A New Era for Bioethics: The Source of Meaning in Moral Experience," in *Religion and Medical Ethics: Looking Back, Looking Forward*, ed. Allen Verhey (Grand Rapids, MI: Eerdmans, 1996), 96–119.

4. Tom Beauchamp and James Childress, *Principles of Biomedical Ethics*, 5th ed. (New York: Oxford University Press, 2001).

5. On the condition of contemporary bioethics, relative to a lack of questioning about moral meaning see Leon Kass, *Life, Liberty and the Defense of Dignity: The Challenge for Bioethics* (San Francisco, CA: Encounter Books, 2002), esp. 55–76; and Gilbert C. Meilaender, *Body, Soul, and Bioethics* (Notre Dame: University of Notre Dame Press, 1955).

6. Alasdair MacIntyre, *Dependent Rational Animals* (Chicago: Open Court, 1999).

7. For a different approach, see Jacob Rendtorff and Peter Kemp, *Basic Principles in European Bioethics and Biolaw*, vol. 1, *Autonomy, Dignity, Integrity, and Vulnerability* (Copenhagen, Neth.: Center for Ethics and Law, 2000), esp. 45–56.

8. See Emanuel Levinas, *Totality and Infinity: An Essay on Exteriority* (Pittsburgh, PA: Duquesne University Press, 1969). For an assessment of Levinas's thought, see Richard Cohen, *Ethics, Exegesis, and Philosophy: Interpretation after Levinas* (Cambridge: Cambridge University Press, 2001). Also, Paul Ricoeur, *Oneself as Another*, trans. Kathleen Blamey (Chicago: University of Chicago Press, 1992); Jean Luc Marion, *Prolegomena to Charity*, trans. Stephen E. Lewis (New York: Fordham University Press, 2002).

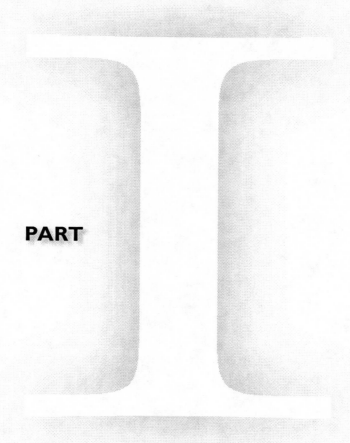

PART

Questioning at the Boundary

Theological Anthropology and Bioethics

Roberto Dell'Oro

This chapter provides a general framework for understanding the contribution of theological anthropology to bioethics. The underlying presumption is that a theological contribution, in bioethics or any other field, requires of the theologian a personal commitment to a particular faith tradition—Roman Catholic in my case—but also openness to the conditions of universal moral communication beyond the limits of one's specific theological affiliation.

Traditionally, the scientific articulation of moral theology has reflected a twofold concern: one for the internal coherence of the theological system, the other for the integration of new philosophical perspectives, in critical dialogue with both culture and society.[1] The success of this methodological program depends, minimally, on two factors: first, a disposition of intellectual generosity on the part of the theologian, namely, his or her willingness to partake in the ongoing reflection of a given community of moral discourse, and second, an attitude of active receptivity on the part of the public the theologian is addressing. A disposition to listen is more than a pure theoretical stance, it is a moral attitude, itself defined by openness to the surprise of meaning coming from unsuspected distances.

At present, the field of bioethics seems to exhibit a certain resistance to the integration of theological voices, a methodological "closure" of sorts that might appear as both unexpected and startling to an attentive observer of the field's beginnings.[2] Bioethics is a relatively new field of study characterized by an interdisciplinary approach to ethical questions raised by advances in biotechnologies and the life sciences. Because of its inherent complexity, bioethics relies upon the contribution of different points of view on the issues it faces. Thus the interaction of theology, philosophy, sociology, and public policy has contributed to a richer understanding of the implications of medical research for society at large. However, whereas thirty years ago the positive contribution of theologians would have been acknowledged as important,[3] it might be met now with an attitude of skeptical resignation.

I argue that the "marginalization" of theological voices in the field of bioethics depends on the convergence of two factors involving, respectively, philosophical and theological ethics. Struggling to find a specific methodology for the dialogue across different disciplines, bioethics tends to reduce the contribution of philosophical ethics to the reconstruction of the conditions for moral consensus in society at large. Although bioethics encounters questions of ultimate meaning as it investigates issues such as genetic engineering, assisted reproductive technologies, euthanasia and assisted suicide, to name but a few, it fails to address these questions' broader ethical significance. Viewing moral pluralism as an obstacle toward the sharing of any "thick" notion of the good within society, bioethics expunges as philosophically uninteresting any attempts to ground such notions on a coherent anthropological basis. In so doing, it replaces questions of moral meaning with questions of procedure and reduces the task of ethics to a logical analysis of moral argumentation, one that functions meaningfully as long as it remains within the framework of a "thin" common morality.[4]

The distinction between "thin" principles of common morality and "thick" notions of the good in bioethics mimics the wider theoretical strategy pursued by political liberalism. For the latter, ethics cannot rationally justify "ideologies of human fulfillment" with their relative notions of the "good life." At best, it can provide criteria for the positive interaction of individual autonomous agents within a community of moral discourse.

Insofar as those criteria are the result of consensual agreement, they can exert normative force only in relation to the *rightness* of the actions they prescribe.[5] However, the *goodness* of the ends implicitly pursued by these actions, the kind of moral personalities and moral societies they yield, remain beyond the scope and limits of ethics.[6]

To such an understanding of the meaning of ethical reflection there corresponds a failure on the part of theological ethics to credibly articulate the *public* relevance of moral insights grounded in the faith experience of religious communities and traditions.[7] Such a failure is particularly visible in the field of bioethics. For here, rather than challenging the prevailing methodological narrowness, theologians either "suspend" their anthropological presuppositions so as to enter the community of moral discourse from a position of neutrality (what Thomas Nagel rather sarcastically calls "a view from nowhere") or become resigned to any possibility of dialogue by claiming for themselves a particularity that is impervious to public criteria of epistemic control and moral interpretation.[8]

In the first part of this chapter, I will address the general cultural condition that feeds into such a predicament and the consequences it forces upon the relation between theology and bioethics. In the second and third parts, I will address the specific question of theological anthropology, relative to the formal aspects of theological anthropology and to its content.

Bioethics and the Postmodern Condition

The cultural situation of our time might be characterized as a condition of fundamental dispersion. The fragmentation of knowledge and the incredible amount of information now available in each discipline make it impossible for anyone to master but a limited amount of material. As a result, we have come to simply accept the limited space of recognized notions and partial perspectives that amounts to our definition of reality, and to feel comfortable within the familiar walls of specialized, yet windowless monads. To put it in the words of Karl Popper, "we are prisoners caught in the frameworks of our theories, our expectations, our past experiences, our language."[9]

Such an atmosphere of epistemological incommensurability is certainly due to the growing complexity internal to each science and appears to be more puzzling in a field like bioethics. Postmodernity is the category currently used to label this complexity. In its broad and, at times, equivocal implications, postmodernity points to a general mood, or *Stimmung*, to borrow the suggestive interpretation of Richard Bernstein.[10] In terms of content, postmodernity entails the definitive overcoming of the modern philosophical and scientific agenda characterized by the optimism of reason and the recognition of a structural fragmentation that, forcing us to the inevitability of contextual interpretations, defies any illusion of totality and, with it, any meaningful pursuit of truth.

The theoretical indeterminacy of postmodernism as a philosophical label contrasts with the clear dimensions of the problems it creates in practice. Two are particularly important and worthy of reflection. First is the problem of bringing together the plurality of lived moralities, what we call moral pluralism, under the common denominator of a shared ethos, or a "common morality" in bioethical jargon. The second is the difficulty of finding a level of discourse that engages differences among moral traditions on questions of substance. Whereas the former problem concerns the moral climate that structures all practical spheres of reality, the latter pertains, more specifically, to the possibility of a theoretical reconstruction of such a moral climate in terms of both ethical discourse and public policy.

Referring to an analysis of different typologies of moral argumentation, MacIntyre observes, "debate between fundamentally opposed standpoints does occur; but it is inevitably inconclusive. Each warring position characteristically appears irrefutable to its own adherents; indeed in its own terms and by its own standards of arguments it *is* in practice irrefutable. But each warring position equally seems to its opponents to be insufficiently warranted by rational arguments."[11]

A way of solving this predicament is to bridge the gap of cultural fragmentation and the unconvincing nature of arguments between moral agents by surreptitiously reducing ethics to a purely regulatory task, thus progressively diluting the distinction between the legal and the moral. The tendency to sublate ethics under the law rests upon the assumption that dialogue on moral convictions separates people; only the law, now invested with a kind of soteriological function, can bring moral differences under the banner of unifying social rules.

I believe such a notion of ethics not only discourages meaningful exchange across different traditions but actually entails, in the long run, a neutralizing effect upon the *content* of moral conversation as such. An ethical discourse capable of mapping out a territory of discussion, where differences can meet and confront each other, will be expunged from the theoretical agenda of ethics. This agenda will, at best, provide a grammar of procedural conditions through which differences among moral traditions may coexist, without ever coming into contact with one another. Rather than focusing on questions of intrinsic value—either in terms of virtues, goods, or some general moral content for action—moral discussion needs only to articulate rules of reciprocal engagement—the a priori of the communication—that will allow each moral participant to remain in a safely protected, yet totally separated, moral universe.

The solution adopted by H. Tristram Engelhardt in *The Foundations of Bioethics* can be presented as an example.[12] His view is based on the conviction that no particular moral vision can provide the ground for a moral consensus. Rational arguments in favor of an ethics of the good, the restoration of a particular framework of moral principles, or the recommendation of a defined set of values would inevitably exacerbate the conflict of opposite interpretations rather than establish the conditions for a peaceful community. As a result, the task of bioethics should be understood "as a disclosure, to borrow a Kantian metaphor, of a transcendental condition, a necessary condition for the possibility of a general domain of human life and of the life of persons generally."[13] Given its regulatory function, bioethics cannot logically predetermine the language of common morality by surreptitiously favoring a particular content over another. The language of bioethics has to be neutral, the "lingua franca" of a society concerned with health care, but incapable of converging around a common viewpoint.

Later in his book, such an ethical formalism becomes even clearer when Engelhardt defines the task of bioethics as "a disclosure of the minimum grammar involved in speaking of blame and praise with moral strangers, and for establishing a particular set of moral commitments with an authority other than through force."[14]

One might accuse Engelhardt of reducing the function of transcendental rationality, with respect to the realm of morality, to the function of an abstract rational agreement as a condition of possibility for the existence of social rules. After all, there is nothing in the nature of this a priori condition that tells us why these rules should be considered specifically moral. In fact, according to Engelhardt, such formalism does not exhaust the whole story of ethics. Its simply defines its "secular" profile, the logical, that is, rational constraints based on the respect for the autonomy of the moral agents involved in moral discourse, without establishing the correctness of any particular moral sense. The regulative character of "secular" bioethics is to function as the logic of pluralism, as the means that will allow the peaceful negotiations of moral intuitions to occur.

Yet, to extend further the Kantian metaphor, if intuitions without concepts are blind, concepts without intuitions remain, for their part, inevitably empty. Thus the question: How can a society retrieve concrete intuitions of the good capable of shaping the moral vision and the conduct of individuals?

Engelhardt's answer to this objection comes in the form of a distinction between community and society. The argument goes like this: on the one hand, *community* designates the free association of individuals through a common and concrete view of the good; *society*, on the other hand, denotes the association of individuals who might pursue a number of important goals together, yet do not share that common vision. The nature of society is essentially pragmatic: it sets forth the conditions for building a limited consensus, one that does not exist, yet needs to be fashioned in order for society to function as a tapestry of different moral communities.

The distinction between society and community translates de facto into the separation between the reasonable claims of a general secular society open to rational control and verification and the theoretical indeterminacy of moralities upheld by particular moral communities, by definition impervious to objective criteria. In the end, the paradoxical situation of moral discourse becomes one of structural fluctuation between a kind of moral rationalism, on the one hand, and dogmatic fideism, on the other. As a fluctuation that entails not only a logical contradiction but also an obvious methodological schizophrenia, it favors a cognitivist presumption for metaethical rationality at the *transcendental* level of society, while reducing the identification with the *categoreal* ethos of a particular community to a pure matter of taste. Indeed, "since there are no generally sustainable, secular arguments to establish as canonical a particular view of the good life and content-full moral obligations, and as long as the ways of life under consideration respect the freedom of the innocent, then, from outside, the choice among any particular moral community will appear to be similar to an aesthetic choice."[15] In this perspective, the impartial, unprejudiced, and nonculturally biased moral agents whose only interest, when functioning within the realm of society, are the logical strength and force of rational arguments, will suspend any residue of intelligence at the threshold of their moral communities. As it appears, within specific communities one must abandon the hope of ever reconciling the loyalty to a moral vision with the consistency of arguments, the fascination with values and virtues with a truly personal and responsible commitment to them.

In order to overcome the problems posed by our postmodern condition, it is imperative to rethink the meaning and purpose of ethical dialogue across different traditions and within the public realm of secular society. One must move here between the Scylla and Charybdis of a dead end: the reduction of ethical rationality to a purely procedural function of political regulation, and the intellectual impotence toward an incommensurable pluralism that legitimizes the relativity of different points of view. Both solutions would be deadly for the articulation of a theological anthropology in bioethics. If the latter is understood as a purely procedural enterprise, then it must exclude as irrelevant to moral discourse an ethics that attempts to convey a theological meaning. Like any other language dealing with particular moral contents, theological anthropology is ultimately bound to live in a separate limbo, and to make sense for those who already understand it: either dissolve into some lowest common denominator, the parallel of Engelhardt's "minimum grammar" or accept a marginal existence as one interesting, yet purely private option. As David Tracy suggests, "neither alternative is acceptable to anyone committed to the truth of any major religious tradition."[16] It would represent the capitulation of theological thinking to ideological relativism and the subjectification of religious experience to the measure of individual taste.

The contribution of theological anthropology to bioethics represents an expression of the publicness of theology and, moreover, an expression of theology's responsibility in serving the intelligence of faith (*intellectus fidei*) and the vision of the good that it entails. Such a responsibility is relative to the momentous significance of the ethical challenges confronting humankind. Are the intuitions of the good, which define the moral treasure of every great religious tradition, to be dismissed from the public debate as fundamentally irrational, or will they be looked at as a reservoir of meaning and wisdom on what it means to be human?

The Form of Theological Anthropology

Though theological anthropology represents a distinct treatise in the canon of theological disciplines, it is referred to in this context in its more obvious connotation, as the understanding of the human as disclosed by Christian revelation.

It is important to state that such an understanding is not given once and for all, but partakes in the historical nature of revelation itself. For this reason, both the *form* and the *content* of theological anthropology remain constantly open to the task of new philosophical reinterpretations. One might think of how the Christian tradition has been able to progressively assimilate and reshape Platonic and Aristotelian *Denkformen* into the Scholastic system and, moreover, how the neo-Scholastic tradition itself has developed in dialogue with transcendental philosophy, the hermeneutic sciences, and the philosophy of language. This is the general meaning of the "anthropological turning point" in theology. According to Karl Rahner, "theology wants to tell man what he is, and what he still remains even if he rejects the message of Christianity in disbelief. Hence theology itself implies a philosophical anthropology, which enables this message of grace to be accepted in a really philosophical and reasonable way, and which gives an account of it in a humanly responsible way."[17]

For the Christian, truths about the human being are implications of truths about God's free and forgiving self-communication, reaching its eschatological, that is, definitive measure, in the Christ-event. Moreover, Christian morality represents the practical mediation of a renewed anthropological understanding flowing from the encounter with the Christ-event and its "effective history" in the life of the Christian tradition.[18]

The structural correlation between theological anthropology and Christian ethics bespeaks a shift in the primacy of moral discourse: the "invitational" character of an anthropological ideal, the call to share in the fullness of meaning disclosed by a particular teleology of human life, one that is also concretely mediated by models of moral conduct, takes precedence over the prescriptive or normative function of moral discourse.

I believe that the meaning of this intuition, which is central to Christian moral discourse, can be grasped when reflecting on how the communication of moral claims—be they values, ideals, or virtues—takes place through the mediation of normative language. One can recognize the fact that there is a certain phenomenological primacy to the normative language, because this is how we come to face moral claims and learn to structure our response to them. Yet from an ontological point of view, the moral language of rules and norms represent a *derivative* function, secondary to the reality of human interaction and communication on ethical insights and notions of human flourishing. At this level, individuals acquire a moral sense by partaking in the moral experience of a community that expresses moral values and ideals symbolically: the texture of moral narrativity structuring the identity of particular communities will comprise a literary testimony of stories, legends, and myths, but also, and perhaps especially, the practical testimony (action) of concrete moral agents. Against the background of such narratives, norms represent an act of solidarity on the part of the community of communication. Individual moral agents do not make moral choices in isolation; rather they always act *in context*, that is, situated by the standards of a community whose practical *rightness* has been historically mediated. Thus moral norms articulate the lived experience of moral subjects and are measured by the concrete potential of their freedom.[19]

Christian ethics will be concerned only *derivately* with moral norms; in the first place, Christian moral discourse will point to the renewed existential condition of human freedom made possible by God's self-communication (grace). To be "in Christ" (*en Christo*), to use a Pauline expression, is the ontological condition for being able to do (to act) like Christ.

It was the particular contribution of the Second Vatican Council to moral theology to stress the importance of such a biblical understanding of moral life, thus overcoming a scholastic version of natural law heavily shaped by the epistemological presuppositions of modern rationalism and the scientific ideal of an ethics *more geometrico demonstrata*. Confront Edwin Healy's conviction, at the beginning of his *Medical Ethics*, that natural law provides the basis for moral principles virtually open to the recognition of every reasonable person: "All men are called upon to obey the natural law. Hence it matters not whether one be a Roman Catholic, a Protestant, a Jew, a pagan, or a person who has no religious affiliation whatsoever; he is nevertheless obliged to become acquainted with, and to observe the teachings of the law of nature. In the present volume all the obligations flow from natural law, unless the contrary is evident from the context."[20]

For the moral theology expressed by the Second Vatican Council the moral life of the Christian should not be conceived as the fulfillment of a previously given impersonal order of natural law, but rather as the response to a call coming from the historical person of Jesus Christ. One can find in some documents of the council a clear evidence of such a Christological approach. For an example, the notion of *sequela Christi* is now referred to as the methodological "structuring principle" of Christian morality.[21] The dialogical structure of the principle brings to bear on moral life the wealth of meaning entailed in the Christian calling to salvation.[22]

Moreover, the theological need to articulate the universal meaning of revelation is not being pursued by sanctioning an essentialist notion of human nature,[23] but rather by articulating the dialectic between the particularity of the Christ-event, with its ethical implications, and the universality of moral experience.

The Christocentric approach of Vatican II helps to shed further light on the distinctive character of moral truth and moral normativity.[24] Moral theology seems to have no particular interest in the theoretical discussion on truth and, as a result, does not seriously confront contemporary theories of truth in order to expand its theoretical tools; it simply finds itself comfortable within the stream of Scholastic tradition. Unfortunately, in so doing, it prevents itself from becoming aware of several difficulties affecting a naïve use of the notion of truth; lacking adequate categories, it falls victim to misunderstandings when it enters into a dialogue with other philosophical positions.

Moral theology relies upon the definition of truth as inherited from the teachings of Aristotle and Aquinas: truth is *adeguatio intellectus et rem*, the conformity of the knowing intellect to its object.[25] This definition conveys an understanding of truth in terms of a formal notion expressing a relation; as such, it presupposes as its condition of possibility the ontological truth of things, itself dependent on God's creative knowledge. Although certainly not wrong, this definition must be further nuanced when applied to moral truth. Moral truth is, by its very nature, the truth of one's life-project; it demands from the person a commitment, the ability to think of one's life and the objectives of one's actions as the result of a practical disposition.

This also sheds some light on the peculiarity of moral reason. Moral reason is not simply predetermined by its object, rather, it is dynamic in that it continually probes and discovers new possibilities. In this way, the goals and objectives for life and action are uncovered and evaluated in light of freedom. Truth does not disclose itself to a purely passive knowledge; instead, knowledge itself exercises an active, constitutive function toward truth.

Moreover, knowledge has a projectlike character that cannot be fully actualized by the individual, but only by an intersubjective, communal engagement. Although it remains true that *consensus non facit veritatem*—consensus does not make truth—it is nevertheless important to recognize that moral experience intermediates the historical meaning of values and ideals relative to a specific life-word with its interpretive framework. Standards of moral performance are gained historically through a process of testing within a community of moral discourse in which all the participants bring to the table their own contribution, in a spirit of freedom and fairness. Theoretical presuppositions must be disclosed in order to exclude positions that ground their claim on the basis of privilege or other uncontrollable sources and to insure the best results in terms of intellectual honesty and transparency.

Borrowing such insights from a consensus theory of truth (see Habermas) might be very important for moral theology, for example, in helping to reshape the notion of *consensus fidelium*. Since moral knowledge is structurally bound to freedom, it represents already the result of a moral performance; hence the paradigm of empirical knowledge falls too short to adequately grasp the very essence of the moral phenomenon.

The relativity of moral truth to freedom must be properly understood, for here freedom does not denote moral choice in its empirical facticity but rather a fundamental willing that constitutes the ontological condition for the possibility of each concrete and free choice. Following the lead of moral theologians schooled in the tradition of Rahner's transcendental theology, one might define *transcendental* freedom as the radical disclosure or self-affirmation of the original will that grounds and sustains empirical freedom.[26] In its dynamic actualization (*Vollzug*), however, freedom is not pitted against its own metaphysical and, ultimately, theological ground, as in the Kantian version of autonomy, but rather it is released to its own identity as love. Each moral decision can be considered good insofar as it mediates the transcendental ground of love upon which it rests; thus each human decision articulates, in a historical way, the radical openness (*Vorgriff*) of human freedom to its own fulfillment (*finis ultimus*).[27]

If the moral norm is relative to freedom, then, it is possible to conclude, without misunderstanding, that the former does not stand over and against transcendental subjectivity as a heteronomistic category. Every moral claim is an expression of the moral agent's autonomy: the person is *in himself or herself* by nature, but becomes *for himself or herself* through the exercise of freedom. Moral experience will be understood as the journey (*ex-perior*) of becoming oneself fully, a journey whose destination cannot be reached without trials and tribulation (*peiros*). In a profound sense, we *are* our freedom, in the sense that our own essence (*actus primus* in Scholastic terms) can be understood only in the act of a radical openness to the reality of being as grace, which calls us to love (see Rahner).

A transcendental hermeneutic of person in terms of freedom represents a definitive overcoming of the traditional notion of person as *rationalis naturae individua substantia*.[28] Person, or personhood, is not to be defined in light of substantialist categories, but rather in terms of process categories, as the *act* of self-actualization that finds its completion in love. Shifting from a definition of personhood in terms of substance to one in terms of act entails realizing that the definition of personhood is, ultimately, *practical* rather than theoretical. In *becoming* a person, the moral subject actualizes the athematic openness (*Vorgriff*) to being as good. The meaning of such a position, however, is to represent the very fulfillment of freedom.

Freedom's fulfillment is not without content, that is, it does not take place in a vacuum: freedom finds in the interpretation of "nature" the material conditions that point in the direction of its telos. In this sense, the classical notion of natural law can be reinterpreted in terms of the law of the person: natural norms are relevant only insofar as they mediate the person's practical destination.[29] *Material*, that is, nonformal universal binding principles of natural law, are grounded in an inductive process of discovery whereby the meaning of fundamental human good is progressively recognized and appropriated as essential to the realization of personal identity. From a transcendental perspective, the objectivity of natural law is thus reduced to transcendental subjectivity. Moral norms of natural law owe their normative force to freedom because they serve the *true* fulfillment of freedom: "Human beings learn by reflecting on their own reactions in the face of challenging demands. In this way, the concept of moral value can be concretized within one's own *experienced* context. This concretization does not invalidate the universality of values. That which is morally true (*das sittliche Wahre*) is always also that which is possible (*das Mögliche*). But what is possible is grasped through the experience of one's own freedom."[30]

In its deepest meaning, however, moral experience is for Christian anthropology an experience of transcendence, relative to the epiphany of an absolute good in the midst of history. To use William Desmond's language, the experience of the good is *metaxological*, because as humans we are given over to the between, a between we do not first create, within which we find ourselves, though we never completely become masters of ourselves or the between. To be ethical is to be in the milieu of the good, between the conditional goods we find and create in the web of relativities, and the unconditional good that is shown or intimates itself in the happening, and to whose promise we respond in the lives we live.[31]

The original mediation of the Christ-event by the primitive community, in terms of both narrative and speculative Christology, speaks to the faith in the disclosure of God's final revelation as the disclosure of an unconditional good for humankind. Such a disclosure is both reassuring and unsettling; on the one hand, it speaks to the depth of human freedom and to its ability to recognize the promise of the good intimated in the Christ-event. At the same time, it speaks of a judgment on the tension experienced by freedom to make the experience of the good into a self-serving project rather than an experience of personal and social liberation.

The experience of the good is, for the New Testament, an experience of love in the sense of both a subjective and an objective genitive. By that,

I mean an experience of being loved, absolutely, which itself grounds the ability to respond to the Other in its radical alterity. The experience of love is an experience of transcendence because the Other is willed in its otherness, irreducible to my needs, my fulfillment, my sense of lack. Moral experience is, in this sense, a response to what is intrinsically valuable and must be affirmed for itself.

Emanuel Levinas has provided great insights for understanding the call of moral experience, the call of the Other, as an *exodus*, an experience of coming out of oneself toward the Other.[32] He also understands that the relation between self and other must shift ontologically (I should say metaphysically) in favor of the primacy of the Other. The Other, mortal and aging, suffers, therefore I am commanded in my singularity, and so commanded, ordered to my singular responsibility for the other all the way, right up to the possibility of dying for the other. Such is for Levinas the nobility, the dignity of the human. That one can be called upon to die for the other, would be the ultimate testimony of a *responsible* self. Thus for Levinas the self is not first for itself and then for the other. Rather, the self rises to its true humanity, to its irreplaceable singularity as an *election*. One is chosen before one chooses. One is oneself when, and insofar as, one is for the other, for the other before oneself.

This might be reformulated in terms of a demystification of autonomy. Freedom released to its own true self in love shows that there is a freedom beyond autonomy. "There is an ethics of the other in which being for the other becomes a free service for the good of the other, a service beyond the calculative self-interest of utilitarian prudence, beyond the determination of autonomous will. We could call this *agapeic* service, a service that serves the good of the other out of a release of freedom towards the other, a release that is an overflow of generosity."[33]

The Content of Theological Anthropology

The contribution of theological anthropology to the public articulation of moral discourse directly flows from the content of faith, understood here as *fides quae*. Klaus Demmer speaks in this context of the maieutic function of faith in relation to moral reason.[34] Although one might encounter within moral theology different interpretive models of the relation between faith and moral reason, it remains undisputable that faith generates a particular anthropological preunderstanding.[35] Faith elicits reflection from moral reason and inspires moral reason. In doing so, it produces in the believer a *specific* horizon of meaning, something like a "system of anthropological coordinates" from which one sees himself or herself and the world. Hermeneutic philosophy has articulated the notion of horizon to define "the range of vision that includes everything that can be seen from a particular vantage point."[36]

The first element in the Christian horizon of meaning is the intrinsic *dignity* of the human person, which is at the root of the principle of autonomy. It flows directly from faith in a personal God as creator, who posits the human being as the event of a free, unmerited and forgiving, and absolute self-communication of God. The Christian tradition has constantly expressed such an understanding of the human being as the image of God, who participates in the new creation of Jesus Christ. Closely connected to this is the awareness of the singularity of one's existence as well as the unrepeatable nature of one's personal history.

This first anthropological implication of faith opens up a special understanding of the uniqueness of each person, of her absolute singularity and incommunicable mode of existing. Though many human beings have existed in the course of history, or are now existing, every person is, as it were, the only one. Every person is a *universale concretum*—a concrete whole—in which there is certainly included the nature of the species with its general characteristics, but also in such a way that this nature is appropriated by the subject in an absolutely singular way, so as to transcend that nature. Thus Romano Guardini defines the singularity of the person as "the fact that she exists in the form of 'belonging to herself' (*in der Form der Selbsgehörigkeit*)."[37]

Creation represents only the beginning of God's self-communication. The Christian God, unlike the Aristotelian first principle, does not limit itself to a position of preeminence in the causal order of beings. God's relation to human history is, in the Christian faith, one of self-communication and complete solidarity. The Christ-event represents the radical and definitive symbol of God's willingness to enter in a communion of love with humankind.

This theological insight opens up new possibilities of meaning in the moral realm at different levels. First, the historical event of the incarnation further articulates the notion of human dignity at an interpersonal level. The fact that God becomes man in the person of Jesus Christ lays the foundation for a radical equality among all human beings and for the notion of social solidarity. Faith indicates that to be in the service of others, especially the most vulnerable and poor, is the very truth of our being-in-the-world with others.

Second, the quality of human history becomes a consideration. Because God shared in the very depth of history, no individual event or dimension of the human experience can be considered, in principle, meaningless. Particularly the experience of suffering remains open to the dimension of hope in light of Christ's death and resurrection, rescued from a final judgment of absurdity and nonsense. Furthermore, the Easter event provides a key to interpreting one's death with all its historical anticipation. If death is not to be the definitive human and moral catastrophe, but rather a passage into a situation of definitive communion with God, then there can be no historical situation that stands outside of this promise and its power to transform.

Some Applications

These are only some of the elements defining the content of theological anthropology, what I have termed an anthropological system of coordinates. Its relevance to specific ethical issues cannot be determined a priori: it requires further steps accompanying the unrelenting work of practical reason.[38] To exemplify the main components of this process, which is both deductive and inductive, consider the belief in the goodness of all creation that informs the Christian attitude toward life. Since the dawn of the Christian tradition, this belief has translated into a new attitude of respect for the poor, the sick, and children, that is, in the unequivocal recognition of their personal status.

This anthropological presupposition, however, needs to be further unpacked in its specific ethical meaning. Thus it is the function of practical reasoning and moral experience to interpret and articulate the ethical implications of such preunderstanding. General moral principles later developed by the Christian tradition, such as the principle of stewardship, or the notion of sanctity of human life, might be seen as plausible inferences of such faith hermeneutics. In their general meaning, however, these principles need to be "specified" in categoreal norms of action through a risky process of ethical justification. One can see that the norm prohibiting the "direct killing of the innocent" stands, for certain, in the effective history of the anthropological a priori mentioned earlier; it represents, nevertheless, the result of a formal process of argumentation not immediately deducible from that a priori. The same holds for the problem of whether it is ethical, in light of the basic tenets of theological anthropology, to experiment on human embryos. The notion of sanctity of human life cannot by itself yield a specific moral norm on the issue. Such a norm will emerge also from weighing the different pre-moral goods involved, that is, from the process of moral reasoning itself.

The system of anthropological coordinates stands at the edge of Christian theology, mediating between theological affirmations and moral norms. Also, it stands as a positive contribution to the public discourse of bioethics, on the presupposition that the public realm is not just a neutral space to be conquered or won over and that the participants in the community of discourse of an "open society" are not to be faced as enemies but as partners. To acknowledge such an a priori of communication of both epistemic and moral relevance has nothing to do with relativism: in fact, dialogue between moral agents, whether "strangers" or "friends," to use the distinction *in vogue*, can only function on the presumption that any claim to meaning and truth be, at the same time, an attestation of freedom and respect for the other. The public realm, as we know all too well, is not an *ideal* community of discourse, but one that is historically determined; thus, it can become subjected to mechanisms of reduction and alienation. In a situation where technology and the market forces have so great a role in molding and transforming our intuitions, feelings and visions of the good for human beings, even reasons and arguments can become merely technical, reflecting strategies for the achievement of goals whose value is measured by an instrumental rather than a specifically moral criterion.

As an example of this process of instrumentalization in the public realm, consider the discussion on stem cell research and the attempt to pit the value of the embryo against the health of so many people who could theoretically benefit from the development of new therapies. This seems the most obvious way to frame the moral quandary in question because, on the one hand, the promises of such a research are so great and, on the other, spare embryos from in vitro fertilization clinics are usually slated to be discarded anyway. Theological traditions will be neatly divided along the line of those favoring a deontological defense of the embryos' moral status as deserving the full respect of persons, and those who will deny such an attribute in favor of a more consequentialist strategy, ready to sacrifice embryos on the basis of something like a utilitarian calculus. Rhetorically, that division will be framed in terms of a clash between conservatives and liberals, the former concerned with the rights of the embryo to life, the latter with the expectations of sick people and the promise of scientific progress.

In reality, the alternative is not so pristine and obvious as it appears. In a closer scrutiny, the discussion can be framed in terms of the alternative described earlier, if one accepts the premises of what is at stake in the comparison, for example, that embryos can be "quantified" and directly measured in the utilitarian calculus against the sum total of health benefits potentially gained from their destruction. But isn't the notion of respect, which everyone agrees the embryo still deserves, what precludes, at least in principle, the possibility of such a direct quantification? The question of the moral status of the embryo is, in itself, a very legitimate and central one for the Christian tradition. However, there might be more. I believe a better look at the system of anthropological coordinates would uncover concerns for the embodiment of the human being as a self, the intrinsic relationality of the person as it extends to issues of justice and distribution. One wonders, and not on theological grounds alone, why the moral argument calling for what has been termed a "policy of small sacrifices" favoring the destruction of embryos should not be invoked in pushing society toward a more just health care system, affordable to everyone, and with obvious beneficial consequences for so many. After all, one could argue, fairness does call for those who have more to make small or big sacrifices for those who have less, or nothing at all. Perhaps somebody may have specific interests in making the public believe that to buy into an "instrumental" way of reasoning means ipso facto to be open mindedly proscience and pro-cure.

To look at the moral arguments of theological anthropology is to realize that they do not stand in isolation, but rather as articulations of an ultimate vision of the good for human beings. I believe, it is the synthetic meaning of this vision as it unfolds in the plurality of theological resources embedding specific moral arguments that is worth interpreting in the public realm. The contribution of theological anthropology is like a thorn in the side of public moral convictions, the source of an unrelenting hermeneutic of suspicion inspired by prophetic courage more than indulgence in post-Cartesian doubt. Courage directs the public discussion in bioethics to the suspension of preconceived judgments and dogmatisms of any kind, making possible the "fusion of horizons" that opens our eyes to a deeper vision of who we are and what is good for us as humans.

NOTES

1. Klaus Demmer, "Das Selbsverständnis der Moraltheologie," in *Grundlagen und Probleme der heutigen Moraltheologie*, ed. Wilhelm Ernst (Würzburg: Echter, 1989), 9–25.

2. Stephen E. Lammers, "The Marginalization of Religious Voices in Bioethics," in *Religion and Medical Ethics: Looking Back, Looking Forward*, ed. Allen Verhey (Grand Rapids, MI: Eerdmans, 1996), 19–43. The perception of a certain resistance to theological perspectives is registered not only in the Anglo-American context. For an example, see Hubert Doucet, "Un théologien dans le débat en bioéthique," *Le Supplément* 202 (1997): 17–37. Also the exchange between Doucet and James J. Walter, "How Theology Could Contribute to the Redemption of Bioethics from an Individualist Approach to an Anthropological Sensitivity," in *CTSA Proceedings* 53 (1998): 53–71.

3. Earl E. Shelp, ed., *Theology and Bioethics: Exploring the Foundations and Frontiers* (Dordrecht: Kluwer Academic Publishers, 1985).

4. Kevin Wm. Wildes, *Moral Acquaintances: Methodology in Bioethics* (Notre Dame, IN: University of Notre Dame Press, 2000).

5. See John Rawls, *A Theory of Justice* (Cambridge, MA: Harvard University Press, 1971); also Jürgen Habermas, *Moral Consciousness and Communicative Action* (Cambridge, MA: MIT Press, 1991) and Habermas, *Justification and Application: Remarks on Discourse Ethics* (Cambridge, MA: MIT Press, 1993).

6. For a critical assessment of this situation in contemporary moral philosophy, see Bernard Williams, *Ethics and the Limits of Philosophy* (Cambridge, MA: Harvard University Press, 1985), esp. 22–70.

7. Lisa Sowle Cahill, "Theology and Bioethics: Should Religious Traditions Have a Public Voice?" *The Journal of Medicine and Philosophy* 17 (1992): 263–72.

8. For an alternative approach, see Dena Davis and Laurie Zoloth, *Notes from a Narrow Ridge: Religion and Bioethics* (Hagerstown, MD: University Publishing Group, 1999).

9. Karl Popper, "Normal Science and Its Dangers," in *Criticism and the Growth of Knowledge*, ed. Imre Lakatos and Alan Musgrave (Cambridge: Cambridge University Press, 1970), 56.

10. Richard Bernstein, *The New Constellation: The Ethical-Political Horizon of Modernity/Postmodernity* (Cambridge, MA: MIT Press, 1992), 59.

11. Alasdair MacIntyre, *Three Rival Versions of Moral Enquiry: Encyclopedia, Genealogy, and Tradition* (Notre Dame, IN: University of Notre Dame Press, 1990), 7.

12. H. Tristram Engelhardt, *The Foundations of Bioethics*, 2nd ed. (New York: Oxford University Press, 1996). His more recent *The Foundations of Christian Bioethics* (Lisse: Swets and Zeitlinger, 2000) does not alter his original view; in fact, it represents the logical articulation of his system in response to the question of the place of religious traditions vis-à-vis secular bioethics.

13. Engelhardt, *Foundations of Bioethics*, 70.

14. Ibid.

15. Ibid., 75.

16. David Tracy, *The Analogical Imagination: Christian Theology and the Culture of Pluralism* (New York: Crossroad, 1981), xi.

17. Karl Rahner, *Foundations of Christian Faith: An Introduction to the Idea of Christianity*, trans. William V. Dych (New York: Seabury Press, 1978), 25.

18. Klaus Demmer, "Moralische Norm und theologische Anthropologie," *Gregorianum* 54 (1973): 263–305.

19. Klaus Demmer, *Leben in Menschenhand: Grundlagen der bioethischen Gesprächs* (Freiburg: Herder, 1987), 31–32.

20. Edwin F. Healy, *Medical Ethics* (Chicago: Loyola University Press, 1956), 7.

21. *Optatam Totius*, 16.

22. Richard McCormick, *The Critical Calling: Reflections on Moral Dilemmas Since Vatican II* (Washington, DC: Georgetown University Press, 1989).

23. One might see such a paradigm at play in the Baroque Scholastic: for example, in Gabriel Vasquez's notion of "*natura metaphysica et absoluta hominis tamquam regula proxima et homogenea moralitatis.*" According to J. Arntz, such a notion influenced the entire neo-Scholastic tradition. See his "Die Entwicklung des naturrechtlichen Denkens innerhalb des Thomismus," in *Das Naturrecht im Disput*, ed. Franz Böckle (Düsseldorf: Patmos Verlag, 1966), 87–120.

24. On the singularity of moral truth, see Klaus Demmer, "Wahrheit und Bedeutung: Objective Geltung im moraltheologischen Diskurs," *Gregorianum* 81 (2000): 59–99. The general methodological background for such reflections can be found in Demmer, *Moraltheologische Methodenlehre* (Freiburg: Herder, 1989). For an explanation of the theological context, see James Keenan and Thomas Kopfensteiner, "Moral Theology out of Western Europe," *Theological Studies* 59 (1998): 107–35.

25. *De Veritate* q. I a. I.

26. Franz Böckle, *Fundamental Moral Theology* (New York: Pueblo, 1980), 55.

27. On the Thomistic understanding of *finis ultimus,* see James F. Keenan, *Goodness and Rightness in Thomas Aquinas's Summa Theologiae* (Washington, DC: Georgetown University Press, 1992). For a reinterpretation of the notion of *finis ultimus* within contemporary moral theology, see Joseph Fuchs, *Moral Demands and Personal Obligations* (Washington, DC: Georgetown University Press, 1993).

28. For a thorough application of the transcendental approach to fundamental moral theology, see Klaus Demmer, *Sein und Gebot: Die Bedeutsamkeit des transzendentalphilosophischen Denkansatzes in der Scholastik der Gegenwart für den formalen Aufriss der Fundamentalmoral* (Munich: Schöningh, 1971). A recent assessment on Demmer's method can be found in Melanie Wolfers, *Theologische Ethik als hadlungsleitende Sinnwissenschaft: Der fundamentalethische Entwurf von Klaus Demmer* (Freiburg: Herder, 2003).

29. One could see this as a transcendental reinterpretation of the traditional notion of natural law as *debitus ordo ad finem.*

30. Klaus Demmer, "Sittlich Handeln aus Erfahrug," *Gregorianum* 59 (1978): 677.

31. William Desmond, *Being and the Between* (Albany: SUNY, 1995).

32. Especially Emanuel Levinas, *Totality and Infinity: An Essay on Exteriority*, trans. Alphonso Lingis (Pittsburgh, PA: Duquesne University, 1969). On Levinas, see Richard A. Cohen, *Ethics, Exegesis, and Philosophy: Interpretations after Levinas* (Cambridge: Cambridge University Press, 2001).

33. William Desmond, *Ethics and the Between* (Albany: SUNY, 2001).

34. In an analogous way, Charles Curran argues that the doctrinal themes of Creation, the Fall, incarnation, redemption, and eschatology serve as the anthropological framework against which moral reason inspired by faith operates. See Charles E. Curran, *New Perspectives in Moral Theology* (Notre Dame, IN: Fides, 1974), 47–86.

35. I am thinking here, most obviously, of the different assessments of the analogy of faith and reason between Catholic and Reformed theologies, but also of the polarity within the Catholic moral tradition itself between an "autonomous morality in a context of faith" and "an ethics of faith." For an overview of the debate, see Vincent MacNamara, *Faith and Ethics: Recent Roman Catholicism* (Dublin: Gill and Macmillan, 1985); also Réne Simon, *Fonder la Morale: Dialectique de la Foi et de la Raison Pratique* (Paris: Seuil, 1974), and Ernst Gillen, *Wie Christen ethisch handeln und denken: Zur Debate um die Autonomie der Sittlichkeit im Kontext katholischer Theologie* (Würzburg: Echter, 1989).

36. Hans Georg Gadamer, *Truth and Method* (New York: Continuum, 1994), 302. For an application of the notion of "horizon" in moral theology, see James J. Walter, "What Can Horizon Analysis Contribute to the 'Consistent Ethic of Life'?" in *The Consistent Ethic of Life: Future Explorations*, ed. Thomas Nairn (Lanham, MD: Sheed & Ward, forthcoming).

37. Romano Guardini, *Welt und Person: Versuche zur christilichen Lehre von Menschen* (Würzburg: Werkbund Verlag, 1955), 128.

38. For an example of how the hermeneutic of faith presuppositions influence the judgments on a concrete moral issue, see James J. Walter, "Human Germline Therapy: Proper Human Responsibility or Playing God?" in *Design and Destiny: Religious Views on Human Germline Modification*, ed. Ronald Cole-Turner (Cambridge, MA: MIT Press, forthcoming).

2

Vulnerability, Agency, and Human Flourishing

Alisa L. Carse

Introduction: The Challenge

Vulnerability is an endemic feature of human life. In this respect we are
not, at one level, distinctive. Like inanimate objects or artifacts, plants,
and nonhuman animals, we can be worn down, broken, lost, or forgotten. Like all living things, both sentient and nonsentient—trees, bees,
flowers, and elephants—we need nourishment, are challenged by disease,
and perish. And like many nonhuman animals—dogs, baboons, dolphins,
cats—we are dependent, social creatures who like to play, who are sensate
and emotional, who are capable of suffering not only adverse conditions
(e.g., of temperature, pollution, malnutrition, disease, ravaging storms) but
also internal states of fear, confusion, and stress. We share with animals a
susceptibility to, in Lisa Sowle Cahill's vivid words, "the vicious, violent,

selfish, and destructive" acts of others.[1] Yet as humans we are also susceptible to committing acts of viciousness, violence, selfishness, and intentional destruction. That is, we are responsible agents, capable of moral and immoral conduct. This fact is tied to, among other things, our capacity for self-reflection and evaluative inquiry, to our ability to act on the basis of value judgments we make, purposes to which we deliberately commit. These capacities render us distinct in the universe of creatures. And this distinctness invites us to examine forms of vulnerability that are peculiarly human, distinctive ways that vulnerability configures human life and affects human flourishing. It challenges us as well to reflect on the implications for moral virtue and conduct of more realistically acknowledging human vulnerability than we traditionally have, both within preeminent philosophical circles in the Western tradition[2] and within important strains of contemporary culture. It is these issues I wish to explore here.

A crucial dimension of our distinctively human predicament is our *dignitary vulnerability*. We are creatures who are susceptible to dignitary struggle: we can be shunned, mocked, dishonored, and subjected to contempt, aversion, and indifference in ways that deeply challenge our sense of value and respect-worthiness, sometimes in spite of our efforts to remain immune, to take "the high road." Persistent devaluation or sustained mistreatment can concretize the degradation of our status. When this happens, human reality falls short of what morality demands. Often we suffer this degradation. But sustained devaluation may render us insensitive to violation, oblivious to disrespect; indeed, it is often a condition of diminished self-respect, a sign of an insufficiently vital and motivating sense of our own intrinsic value and worth, that others' devaluations fail to elicit our pain or protest. Yet when we feel degraded and when we don't, being subject to degradation can be profoundly disabling to the confidence, trust, and self-possession required for healthy, effective human agency. Our dignity is a fragile, vulnerable good.

As these comments no doubt suggest, we commonly think of "vulnerability" in a negative sense: to be vulnerable is to be susceptible to loss, "injury[,] and insult."[3] I will here explore a broader understanding of vulnerability, examining ways it is in play in our suffering, our travails, and our thriving. First, it is in many cases precisely those factors essential to human flourishing that render us vulnerable. The loss of a child to illness or the rejection by a beloved can cast us into dark disorientation and pain—states of terrible yearning, grief, or desolation. Yet it is because we so deeply love our child or our friend that we are vulnerable to losing them. Similarly, the creative process confronts us with our vulnerability. Scientific work that demands patient, resilient, long-term commitment will sometimes come to naught. A pianist whose hands are rendered strong and supple through countless hours of devoted practice may lose use of them to arthritis. So too life can be derailed by devastating earthquakes or droughts, made miserable through political tyranny or the deprivation and anxiety imposed by poverty in unjust conditions. It is clear, then, that our flourishing is subject to the vicissitudes of fortune, to disease and disability, to the powers of nature, and to the choices and conduct of others—in short, to a world that is, in many ways, outside our control. But these reflections reveal a second point as well, namely, that while our flourishing can be imperiled by our vulnerability, it also *requires us to be vulnerable*—that is, our flourishing is in crucial ways *constituted by* vulnerability. Being open, receptive, flexible, and tender,[4] being emotionally invested in relationships or committed to undertakings, being capable of nurturing and being nurtured, of loving and growing are necessary to realizing some of the most profound "goods" of human life. Flourishing entails the capacity to let down our guard, relax a rigid agenda-driven orientation, take off our armor, and allow ourselves to be "raw"—exposed in our needfulness, dependency, attachment, and passions. As Aristotle wisely recognized, invulnerability would be—in Martha Nussbaum's words—"purchased . . . at too high a price [in] a life bereft of . . . important values."[5] A life worth living is full of risk.

To acknowledge human vulnerability is to face head-on our finitude, embodiment, profound interdependency, and moral susceptibility in ways that give the lie to a picture that holds us captive—a picture I, invoking a phrase from the philosopher Norman Care, call the "received view," or *myth*, of the "in-control agent."[6] It is, in part, because of our investment in this "myth" that we suffer indignity in illness, feel degraded by dependency, and (at times) react with fear, aversion, and contempt in the face of others' afflictions.

The "In-Control" Agent

It is a fascinating and significant fact that much of philosophical history, notoriously, though not solely, in Western, post-Enlightenment thought,[7] has embraced a view of human agency and the human self that has underplayed our vulnerability. The predominant model of agency in terms of which our flourishing is conceived, and to which dignitary status is attached, is one highlighting self-sufficiency, independence, a capacity for deliberation and rational transcendence of emotion—that is, effective self-determination and self-control, grounded in our capacity as "willers." On this model, we are able to determine our own motivations and conduct on the basis of reasons, freeing ourselves from the forces of fear, desire, anxiety, grief, and the like. This is the dream of autonomy and "invincibility"[8] that has held us captive.

It is true that the myth of the in-control agent does not dominate TV shows or popular music, nor is it a conception generally inspiring literature, drama, or poetry. We tend to find the most compelling dramas in human frailty and failing—in tragic loss and error, unwise romantic surrender, unrequited love and inconsolable yearning, our capacity for envy, fear, and cruelty. But while the in-control agent tends not to inspire art, it creeps into many dimensions of our culture as a "default model"—our practices of praising and blaming, rearing children, designing schools and curricula,[9] and creating the cult of superheroes (now with the indomitable video game warriors that rivet children—e.g., in "SoulCaliber II," "Super Smash Bros. Melee," or "Megaman"). Our standards of attractiveness and success, too, celebrate youth, vigor, and productivity; our adulation of athletes and our notions of strength and leadership center on mastery and control. Moreover, the in-control agent is a conception that informs dominant moral-philosophical paradigms, models, and exemplars—what is seen as morally mature and responsible. It thus represents a benchmark against which our frailties and failings as agents are assessed.

We must not, of course, abandon altogether the values driving this myth, for they guide our condemnation of coercive, tyrannical, and manipulative practices. As Joel Feinberg points out, we do not experience mere "frustration or antipathy" in response to paternalistic constraints or other infringements of autonomy. The "moral indignation and outrage" provoked convey a view that we have been "violated, invaded, belittled."[10] When others attempt to control us in certain ways, this counts as moral disregard; we are treated with insufficient respect. Nonetheless, the myth of the in-control agent is morally costly, for there is much about the human condition that it obscures, ignores, distorts, and effectively denigrates in virtue of its silence about our vulnerabilities. This is what keeps it a myth rather than a meaningful and useful regulative ideal. The challenge is to explore how dignity and effective agency can be respected and sustained in an approach to flourishing that is frank about the limitations of our self-determination and control and the realities of our interdependency.

Human Affliction: The Vicissitudes of Fortune, the Limits of Control

Affliction in all its forms confronts us with the brute limitations of our control over the course our lives take. Illness, disability, and suffering that are intermittent or short lived are more easily integrated into a general sense of competency and independence. By contrast, acute or chronic physical pain, sustained disability or weakness, or the toll of tragic loss and traumatic assault more starkly confront us with our vulnerability and often too with our need for the support and care of others. Life takes many twists that can challenge us, derail us, isolate us from others, and leave us unable, in fact, to cope alone.

First, as much literature emphasizes, a paradoxical relationship to the body often attends bodily affliction. On the one hand, we are confronted vividly with the fact of our embodiment as agents. Pain can rivet our attention, shrinking the compass of our concern to the perimeters of the body; moreover, as bodily demands increase, they often come to occupy much of our conscious focus.[11] Practical agency and identity are more permeated by awareness of our body. On the other hand, in suffering pain or confronting bodily impediment our embodiment can at the same time represent a *threat* to our agency and identity, a source of frustration, loss, and diminution. As Kay Toombs forcefully describes, "the lived experience of bodily breakdown is invariably accompanied by an acute awareness of alienation from one's body"; one is "at its mercy," impotent in the face of its stubborn progress toward further dissolution, pain, "malfunction," even torturous suffering.[12]

Such a paradoxical relationship of the "self" to the body can emerge through both physical illness and disability but also in the wake of violation and assault. Writing of her rape and attempted murder just as she and her husband were joyously trying to conceive a child, Susan Brison notes, "My body was now perceived as an enemy, having betrayed my newfound trust and interest in it, and as a site of increased vulnerability. But rejecting the body and returning to the life of the mind was not an option, since body and mind had become nearly indistinguishable. My mental state (typically depression) felt physiological, like lead in my veins, while my physical state (frequently, incapacitation by fear and anxiety) was the incarnation of a cognitive and emotional paralysis resulting from shattered assumptions about my safety in the world."[13]

Just as bodily affliction can profoundly compromise our flourishing and threaten, even undermine, our sense of self-determination and effective agency, so too can the onslaught of "intrusive" emotional states"—for example, terror, grief, despair, or anxiety.[14] Such states can beset us, "take over," riding free of our will or capacity to control, modulate, or reason our way out of them. "The immediate psychological responses to . . . trauma," Brison writes, "include terror, loss of control, and intense fear of annihilation. Long-term effects include the physiological responses of hypervigilance, heightened startle response, sleep disorders, and the more psychological, yet still involuntary, responses of depression, inability to concentrate, lack of interest in activities that used to give life meaning, and a sense of a foreshortened future."[15] Brison refers to these effects as "autonomy-undermining symptoms" that "reconfigure the survivor's will, rendering involuntary many responses that were once under voluntary control."[16]

This brings me to a second point. Often, in the grip of affliction, particularly when it is chronic or sustained, facets of our identity outside the sources of affliction recede to the background, especially as dependency increases or vital functions are compromised. We *become* the diseased body, the victimized person or "survivor," the "walking wounded," as illness, assault, injury, or grief fix our and others' attention. The fact that one is (or was) a teacher, a firefighter, a kind and gracious neighbor, a deft dancer, a concentration camp survivor, or a "performance artist" becomes increasingly invisible, eroding the ability to sustain one's practical identity in the face of disablement and dependency now dominating life. Thus we suffer "ontological assault"—often accompanied by a sense of powerlessness,[17] and so too by eerie disorientation and keen feelings of mourning. The toll of affliction can draw us away from the fascinations and involvements that once captivated us, informed our core identity, and united us with others in shared pursuits.

Third, one of the ways in which physical and psychic pain induce *suffering* is through the "agony" of isolation.[18] In a public, shared world that blithely proceeds as if illness, death, and trauma do not exist, disease and affliction have no "dignified" place; they are often silently or secretly endured, hidden from view, moved into the privatized, sequestered arenas of the home, the clinic, or lonely awareness.

In part, conditions of pain, disability, weakness, and grief themselves introduce roadblocks to participation in ordinary social activities. Work, play, creative collaboration, and socializing require energy, verve, and stamina.[19] Not only can affliction deplete the energy needed to engage in familiar pursuits, but it can also separate us from a social world oriented around presumptions of bodily strength, emotional endurance, and unaided mobility—often a world that was once "our own."[20] If we live with chronic disability, participation can require relentless ongoing struggle.

The isolation from others is often compounded as well by the felt absence of adequate language with which to communicate our experience to others. Dorothee Soelle writes of the state of "mute suffering": "The weight of unbearable suffering makes us feel totally helpless; we are stripped of the autonomy to think, speak, and act."[21] The sense that our experience defies language or shared, public understanding itself renders us insulated; suffering is exacerbated by our "unspeakable" condition and by the humiliation of our inability to mobilize language to secure the understanding of others and thereby ease the pain of estrangement and isolation. The public celebration of healthful vigor, drive, and ebullience enhances the isolating impact of suffering, its felt incomprehensibility. Recalling his experience at a professional conference following the sudden death of his young wife, Robert Stolorow writes, "as I looked around the ballroom, [the other people] seemed like strange and alien beings to me. Or more accurately, I seemed like a strange and alien being—not of this world. The others seemed so vitalized, engaged with one another in a lively manner. I, in contrast, felt deadened and broken, a shell of the man I had once been. An unbridgeable gulf seemed to open up, separating me forever from my friends and colleagues. They could never even begin to fathom my experience, I thought to myself";[22] "an anguished sense of estrangement and solitude [took] form."[23]

Fourth, and deeply disturbingly, the social isolation of affliction is reinforced by the aversion and contempt it elicits in others. As Simone Weil writes, "Great affliction . . . arouses disgust, horror, and scorn."[24] The well-bodied and thriving often resent and withdraw from those who are suffering or struggling, loath to confront palpable evidence of human vulnerability, and thus their own susceptibility to bodily breakdown, disability, death, or despair. A common theme among rape victims, for example, is the tendency of others to diminish the seriousness of their experience, urging them to "move on" and "get past it." The survivor of assault who "goes public" is often "marked" and stigmatized by the violation she has suffered, viewed as sullied and ruined, and subjected to others' repugnance and avoidance. In efforts to sustain the myth of self-determination and control to which we are so attached, victims are frequently blamed for the violation they endured ("you jogged alone in the dark"; "What were you thinking wearing that low-cut dress?").[25] A parallel tendency accompanies attempts to account for illness by appeal to bad choices in diet or lifestyle, to view the ill as "defective," irresponsible choosers. And when we ourselves are wedded to society's dominant "scripts" of responsible agency, or invested in an identity tied to control, independence, or self-sufficiency, let alone its narrow standards of attractiveness and success, we are susceptible

to shame, humiliation, even horror in becoming sick, experiencing a dissolution of physical strength and independence, or suffering assault or violation. The terrorized aftermath of violent assault is notoriously burdened by
shame on the part of the survivor.[26] So too is the "disfigurement" of disease
or injury. More generally, physical and psychological afflictions *characteristically* induce in those who suffer them "a sense of . . . deficiency,"[27] a
feeling of diminishment and degradation, challenging, even eroding, our
sense of dignity and effectiveness, making us feel "defective."

The question thus arises how, through an honest acceptance of our actual
vulnerabilities, we can succeed in creating forms of human connection in
which our felt sense of dignity and effective agency can be secured and sustained. After all, we do, as human beings, have a distinctive capacity for
interpreting and finding meaning in our experience. Clearly we must abandon a moral orientation in which disability, dependency, and affliction are
understood and experienced as "indignities" signaling deficiency or failure.

Taking Human Vulnerability to Heart

Much suffering that attends human vulnerability is in significant part a
consequence of our attitudes toward our own and others' vulnerabilities.
While there is a lot in life that is inescapably painful, we bring unnecessary pain upon ourselves through entrenched patterns of fear and denial.
In the next paragraphs I explore ways we can take human vulnerability to
heart in the service of human flourishing. In doing so, I will suggest that it
is precisely *in taking our vulnerability to heart*—in embracing rather than
fearing or denying it—that vital forms of human connection, crucial to our
flourishing, are made possible.

In *Rational Dependent Animals*, Alasdair MacIntyre writes:

We human beings are vulnerable to many kinds of affliction and most
of us are at some time afflicted by serious ills. . . . What resources
an individual needs varies with circumstances, temperament, and
above all the obstacles and difficulties that have to be confronted.
We need others to help us avoid encountering and falling victim to
disabling conditions, but when, often inescapably, we do fall victim,
either temporarily or permanently, to such conditions . . . we need
others to sustain us, to help us in obtaining needed, often scarce,
resources, to help us discover what new ways forward there may be,

and to stand in our place from time to time, doing on our behalf what we cannot do for ourselves. . . . [A]t different periods of our lives we find ourselves, often unpredictably, at very different points on [the scale of dependency and need].[28]

It is crucial, first, to recognize that dependency and need form an ineradicable dimension of the human condition; they do not, as such, represent "defective" agency.[29] If we embrace this fact, then we must ask what moral pressure it exerts on us as fellow human beings. I believe that among the many moral implications we might here explore, there are three in particular that emerge as deeply important, namely, *cultivating the virtues of healthy empathy, sustaining compassion toward others*, and *joining in solidarity with those in need*.

Empathy and Compassion

In a compelling analysis contrasting empathy with "detached concern" in physician-patient relationships, Jodi Halpern writes that empathy involves "imagining *how* it feels to experience something, in contrast to imagining *that* something is the case."[30] To engage empathically entails entering a state of "emotional resonance" with another,[31] or, in Adrian Piper's words, "visceral," felt "comprehen[sion] of [another's] condition."[32] Moreover, it engages our imaginations, for we must, as Halpern says, attempt to grasp the "details and nuances of the patient's life" to try to feel our way into her experience of "illness, disability, or psychological injury."[33] It is crucial to imagine the other's condition *in its meaning for her* (as best we can).[34] Along these lines, Nel Noddings characterizes a form of receptive attunement, central to caregiving, that "involves stepping out of one's own personal frame of reference into the other's."[35] As caregiver, she says, "I set aside my temptation to analyze and to plan. I do not project; I receive the other into myself, and I see and feel with the other."[36]

While empathy is an essential element of "compassion," compassion also, as it is often construed, entails a desire to actively alleviate others' suffering or distress. In compassion, the other's condition is "felt," and their welfare is a focus of committed support and concern.

Why the emphasis on empathy and compassion? If affliction is not to erode our sense of intrinsic value and respect-worthiness or utterly to subvert the effectiveness of our agency, we must address the isolation it imposes.

Empathic, compassionate engagement makes it possible for us to forge relational connections even in the face of disabling affliction. They constitute forms of meaningful presence, which are also important to attempts to draw another out of her fortress of insularity so that her felt condition can be grasped and addressed, and—with luck—ultimately integrated without shame into her sense of self and "identity."[37]

Several caveats are crucial here. First, to highlight the importance of empathy and compassion is not to deny that we can, as Lawrence Blum notes, feel "moved" or "'touched' by another's plight . . . without sharing . . . in her distress or suffering."[38] It is important to emphasize, too, that the claim is not that we are to move into an unbounded descent into the state of the other. It is, rather, that effective responsiveness to others often entails forms of emotional attunement and openness that go beyond a mere poignant acknowledgment that another is suffering or in distress. Consider a woman confronting terminal illness who manifests signs of acute anxiety. Imagine that she is a young mother and an accomplished dancer. Perhaps she is afraid she will suffer, or terrified about the prospect of dying. Perhaps her "anxiety" is primarily about the loss of those capacities needed to provide for her children or ever to dance again. She may be gripped by guilt-ridden anticipatory dread about the disruption and grief her illness will bring to her family. She may fear the resentment she imagines others will feel toward her as she becomes increasingly weak and needful, or she may be resentful herself—even furious—about the "unfairness" of being struck down by illness at such a young age. These factors make a difference to how we are effectively to respond in providing the care and support she needs. While we can sometimes rely on simple observations ("She is acutely anxious"), being present to another in a rich and vibrant way, being able to be with her empathically by "getting inside" or "grasping" her felt experience, can be crucial both to a rich *understanding* of her experience and to the particular *expressive* quality of our own presence and intervention, our ability to reach her in the remote place of her affliction. This is an important part of creating the trust needed to help her in recalling valued intimacies or to empower her in beginning to grasp the forms of initiative, competence, and autonomy that her life still permits, thus supporting her movement out of the acute anxiety "freezing" her agency.[39]

Second, it is important, of course, not to be too blithe or sanguine here. In attempts to be empathic, we must guard against the peril of inappropriate involvement—the danger that we might be intrusive in our presence, or, on the other hand, ourselves compromised—"vicarious[ly] possessed"—by the state of the other as we imagine it.[40] While a temporary relaxation of our own perspective or "frame" can serve valuable connection or "resonance," receptivity must not be confused with disrespectful violation of the other's desired privacy or our own submissiveness to a perspective that may be distorted or confused. A properly bounded caregiver must, on the one hand, be sufficiently respectful of and open to another in need while, on the other hand, sustaining the self-possession, emotional equanimity, and critical distance required to avoid unhealthy self-effacement. Moreover, if I am emotionally "infected" by your fear or grief, "filled" with your sense of doom or anxiety, I risk becoming consumed by my own reactive distress, riveted by my own discomfort, and diverted away from the emotional reality of your experience.[41] Unbounded empathic forays can compromise healing connection, undermining compassionate response. Furthermore, our imaginations are limited; we must remain sober about our capacity to actually grasp the other's felt condition. The challenge is to widen and expand our emotional engagement and imaginative power while maintaining proper humility and morally appropriate boundaries.[42]

Effective Agency Reconsidered: The Centrality of Human Connection

The role of empathy and compassion can be illustrated in different kinds of examples. As we have seen, "metabolizing" or integrating our experience of illness and suffering is often difficult. We may be too overwhelmed to articulate our feelings or to express them in publicly accessible language; we may not trust others to understand. It is important, in addressing the isolation of affliction, to acknowledge the value of silent, supportive presence, a presence that sometimes communicates humbleness about the limitations of one's own comprehension at the same time that it conveys invested concern, or again, a presence that conveys respect for the sheer incomprehensibility and disorientation of pain or disablement the other suffers, along with a desire to do what one can to alleviate it.[43] In a discussion of therapeutic relationships, Daniel Siegel characterizes a state of emotional "alignment" that "permits a nonverbal form of communication" to a patient that she is being "felt" by another person.[44] Entering such a state communicates both an attempt to join the other, easing her isolation, and one's hope, in so doing, to ameliorate her suffering. In "feeling felt" in this way, a patient can develop the fledgling sense of trust needed to begin to bridge the seemingly "unbridgeable gulf" Stolorow speaks to, "the sense of estrangement and solitude" that affliction often creates.[45]

Even when language is accessible, the capacity for realistic and flexible reflection can be disabled by the condition of pain or suffering. In her analysis of doctor-patient relationships, Halpern[46] characterizes ways patients become stuck in "concretized" emotional states—so overwhelmed and flooded by "fear, anxiety, despair," that their reflective ability—in particular, "to imagine alternative ways that [they] might feel in the future under varying conditions" is obstructed—that they hold on to a conception of their circumstances that is "unrelenting and immune to genuine reflection."[47] Under such conditions, Halpern argues, the patient's rational reflective abilities (at least concerning her health prospects and medical options) are radically compromised. The role of the physician, she maintains, must exceed the pursuit of "informed consent," simply understood. It must also involve efforts to engage the patient, actively attempting—sometimes through psychiatric intervention, sometimes through sustained compassionate presence and communication—to bring the patient out of rigid isolation, into a condition in which she feels safer, and is hence able to think more flexibly and realistically about her options.[48] In this way, the patient's sense of connection and trust can be enhanced, helping her both to reenter human relationship and to regain effective rational agency—here, making genuine consent, and thus a form of "self-determination," possible.

A common theme, both in trauma literature and in literature on suffering, is the importance of finding language with which to begin to communicate one's experience, to tell one's story to others.[49] Communicative efforts may at first be ones of "lamentation"—expressions of grief and pain, pleas for relief. But, ultimately, the construction of a more articulated narrative that can be heard and understood is imperative to regaining a sense of agency and control, to achieving ownership and integration of one's plight. Brison writes about "moments of reprieve from vivid and terrifying flashbacks [of her assault] when giving [her] account of what had happened—to the police, doctors, a psychiatrist, a lawyer, and a prosecutor," and several years later to a jury that believed her and sentenced her assailant for rape and attempted murder.[50] "Whereas traumatic memories (especially perceptual and emotional flashbacks) feel as though they are passively endured, narratives are the result of certain obvious choices (how much to tell to whom, in what order, etc.)." This in turn helps to reign in memories, to determine when you will be beset by them, "making them less intrusive and giving them the kind of meaning that enables them to be integrated into the rest of life."[51]

The importance to healing of "feeling felt," of others' intervening to ease one out of concretized and frozen states of psychic pain, or of being "heard" in telling one's story all attest to the profound relationality of the self and its role in our capacity to flourish. Such reflections also reveal a form of "control" that is realized, not in simple self-determination or brute independence but in a renewed sense of empowerment through processes of shared exploration; in exercising capacities for mutuality through which we can emerge out of isolation and, ultimately, begin to take initiative in clarifying the particular meaning of our experience—in some cases reorienting our identity to incorporate feelings of pain, limitation, anger, or grief. Exercising "control" in this way entails the creative work of transformation. Undertaking this creative process requires, among other things, trust in the capacity of another (or others) not to abandon us, to sustain "a secure alliance" with us in this risky voyage,[52] and—crucially—to be compassionate in understanding our story and its personal significance.[53]

Empathy and compassion draw on and mobilize a constellation of character traits and excellences—patience; generosity; tender curiosity; humility; and a willingness to remain open in our interpretation of situations, to resist imposing our own interpretations and agendas on others, to invest in the other's well-being, and often to stay the course through rocky terrain. This in turn requires flexibility—as Lawrence Blum puts it—that we remain "alive to the ways that a given situation might differ from others (to which it might be superficially similar) [and] . . . with which it has been correlated (within one's own experience) in the past . . . [or] to which we might otherwise assimilate it."[54] Crucially, all of these virtues and excellences *constitute states of vulnerability*, for they entail relaxing control and allowing ourselves to be affected, risking disappointment, disruption, and sometimes unnerving emotional contact with the pain and loss, the rage and despair, of another. Allowing ourselves to be vulnerable in this way requires courage.

Realizing empathy and compassion is thus no small feat. Disengagement, avoidance, emotional remoteness, indifference, or even callousness are, as we have seen, common responses to affliction, and to the fear and anxiety it can provoke. So too are reactions of aversion and contempt. In addition, the toll and exhaustion of caregiving can create resentment and anger in the caregiver. All such reactions undercut our identification with others in need, constricting the scope of emotional and imaginative resonance. This, in turn, often leads to outright neglect, abandonment, or injury, compounding feelings of isolation, degradation, and shame in those already burdened by suffering and dependency.[55]

Solidarity

These reflections suggest that a realistic acknowledgment of human vulnerability and the challenges it presents takes us beyond the virtues of face-to-face empathy and compassion. If we are to encourage the cultivation of necessary courage and to recognize and significantly allay the burdens and risks of giving and receiving care, we must create a culture accepting of, and responsive to, human finitude and dependency, a culture that supports caregivers and caregiving, and in which it is normal and expected that we join in solidarity with those in need.[56] To this end, it is, as Alasdaire MacIntyre writes, crucial to "envision . . . a form of political society in which it is taken for granted that disability and dependence on others are something that all of us experience at certain times in our lives and this to unpredictable degrees, and that consequently our interest in how the needs of the disabled are adequately voiced and met is not a special interest . . . but rather the interest of the whole political society, an interest that is integral to their conception of their common good."[57]

Achieving the "common good" so construed requires a vital awareness of the vulnerability all of us confront as human beings, and thus a humble identification on the part of each of us with the weal and woe of others. Joining in solidarity with others goes beyond expressions of fellow-feeling to the work of creating practices and institutions responsive to suffering of all kinds—brought by illness, hunger, violence, loss, exclusion, and tragedy. This work addresses not only institutions of the state but "political society" broadly understood,[58] extending into civil arenas of family, school, workplace, hospitals, prisons,[59] and the like. It demands broad and pervasive conditions of mutual respect—a commitment to the equal intrinsic value and respect-worthiness of human beings as such. It also demands positive concern for, and investment in, the thriving of all human beings. This is no small order. The realization of practices embodying mutual respect and concern is threatened by bigotry and hatred, by competitive desires and motivations, and by more seemingly innocuous forms of "tunnel vision" rooted in indifference toward others or ignorance about their plight. It is also, as we have seen, threatened by the many, often unconscious and unacknowledged, aversions and fears that are in fact in play in our resistance to joining with others or taking their legitimate needs to heart, especially when we stand at a distance from them geographically, culturally, or relationally. These attitudes significantly challenge civic virtue in ways so commonplace as to pose a genuine threat to human flourishing that cannot be alleviated through laws and policies. We must strive to combat divisions rooted in fear and indifference and to cultivate virtues of "acknowledged dependency"[60] such as those we have been exploring. Virtues of empathy, compassion, and solidarity must thus work hand in hand.

In endeavoring through shared, reflective commitment to cultivate virtues of human connection and their material expression in our practices and institutions, we encounter a form of responsible agency compatible with an honest, straightforward acceptance of human limitation. This form of responsible agency is not expressed centrally through independence and individual autonomy—although forms of self-control and self-discipline are without question required in stemming the forces of self-absorption and fear. It is expressed most centrally through the committed collaborative work of tending the afflicted and of fighting for inclusive conditions of social justice that do not marginalize those most vulnerable. Such efforts cannot succeed in determining a transformed reality "on a dime," but there is evidence of the power and significance human solidarity has throughout the global human community.[61]

Conclusion

Physical affliction, poverty and deprivation, violent assault at the hands of others, the loss of a loved one, or the destructive forces of nature can wreak havoc in human life, shattering our basic sense of safety and introducing an acute awareness of our own vulnerability—of the unpredictability and contingency of our lives. Our routines can be upset, our aspirations rendered moot, our familiar modes of living brought to a disorienting end. When we are thwarted or "unhinged," our flourishing becomes especially dependent on the support of others, even others with whom we have up until now shared a basic equality of dependency and need. Moreover, asymmetries of dependency and need fundamentally configure many relationships that fill our lives (e.g., in youth or old age, as students or patients, when we are ill or disabled) in ways that are neither "abnormal" nor morally problematic as such. We need the protection and sustenance of others; our flourishing is threatened by others' neglect.

Our attachment to impoverished paradigms of control and self-determination in human life diminishes our potential to join others in meaningful forms of connection essential to human flourishing. Acceptance of our vulnerabilities, when combined with the virtues of empathy, compassion, and solidarity, can ground and motivate a moral call to provide all people with needed forms of sustenance and support—to ameliorate the isolating impact of suffering, to help in the work of "healing" among those facing chronic disability or terminal illness, to sustain contexts in which those left shaky or terrified in the aftermath of trauma can regain trust and self-respect, and—most fundamentally—to ensure minimally decent conditions necessary for the realization and expression of those capacities for evaluative reflection, commitment, and generous-hearted collaboration that mark human beings as unique in the universe of creatures.

Allowing ourselves *to be vulnerable* is necessary to loving and being loved, to caring and being cared for, and to playing, exploring, and growing in ways that strengthen and vitalize our effective agency. Our vulnerability is inextricably tied to our capacity to give of ourselves to others, to treasure and aspire, to commit to endeavors, to care about justice and about our own and others' dignity. Soberly facing the limitations of self-sufficiency and self-determination is a crucial dimension of sustaining (and sometimes regaining) a felt sense of dignity through genuine communion with others in the face of life's unpredictability and risks, its hardships and tragic turns.

NOTES

I presented an early version of this essay at the conference "A Theological Anthropology for Bioethics," Georgetown University, sponsored by The Center for Clinical Bioethics, Georgetown University, November 5–6, 2004. I am grateful to all present for stimulating discussion, from which I learned a great deal. I wish to also extend warm thanks to my father, James Carse, for thoughtful responses to an earlier draft of the chapter, and to Mary Dluhy and Edmund Pellegrino for their inspiration.

1. Cahill, this volume.

2. Alasdair MacIntyre, *Dependent Rational Animals: Why Human Beings Need the Virtues* (Chicago: Open Court Press, 1999) represents a notable exception, which is an inspiration to me.

3. Indeed "vulnerability" derives from the Latin *vulnerare*; to be vulnerable is, in the dictionary definition, quite narrowly to be "capable of being physically wounded," "open to attack or damage: assailable." The phrase "injury and insult" appears in *Webster's Ninth New Collegiate Dictionary*'s entry on "tenderness." See note 4 below.

4. Intriguingly, "tenderness" has a dual meaning important to the view I am exploring here. *Webster's Ninth New Collegiate Dictionary* defines it as, on the one hand, "having a soft or yielding texture: [being] easily broken, cut, or damaged,

delicate, fragile," susceptible to "injury and insult." Yet on the other hand, to be "tender" is to be "respon[sive] to, or express[ive] [of] the softer emotions appropriate or conducive to a delicate or sensitive constitution or character: gentle."

5. Martha Nussbaum, *The Fragility of Goodness: Luck and Ethics in Greek Tragedy and Philosophy* (New York: Cambridge University Press, 1986), 322.

6. In a forceful analysis, Norman Care, "Problematic Agency," in *Living with One's Past* (Lanham, MD: Rowman and Littlefield, 1996), examines factors of "constitutional luck," focusing on "constitutional shyness," "alcoholism," acute depression, and an addiction to the molestation of children, asking to what extent we see these dispositions or conditions as under persons' "control."

7. This conception didn't begin with the Enlightenment, of course. Plato, Aristotle, and Aquinas, among many others, highlight intellect and will as grounding the form of self-determination characteristic of human agents.

8. I take this term from Kay Toombs, who eloquently characterizes dominant culture's measure of "success" in terms of forms of "invincibility" (this volume).

9. David Brooks, "The Organization Kid," *Atlantic Monthly,* April 2001, illustrates this trend in American culture as it informs child-rearing practices. Brooks studies a first-year class at Princeton, arguing that the youth culture at this high end of "success" is characterized by a tenacious reliance on agendas and plans, an avoidance of intimacy or risk, the absence free play, and general isolation from the weal and woe of others on the globe, manifested among other things in relative ignorance about politics and current events. This is, of course, Brooks's reading, which I here present rather than endorse. Whether or not it is true of Princeton undergraduates, my suggestion is that it characterizes a powerful trend among high-performance youths in the United States. In a very different context, Rowan Williams, *Lost Icons: Reflections on Cultural* Bereavement (New York: Morehouse Publishing, 2000), offers a compelling reflection on contemporary understandings of "childhood" (at least in preeminent Anglo-American cultural strains) that fail sufficiently to value the significance of fantasy, play, and playacting as crucial developmental activities.

10. Joel Feinberg, "Autonomy," in *The Inner Citadel,* ed. J. Christman (New York: Oxford University Press, 1989), 27.

11. See M. Therese Lysaught (this volume) for an excellent discussion of this theme. Lysaught draws on the work of B. Hanson, "School of Suffering," in *On Moral Medicine: Theological Perspectives in Medical Ethics,* ed. S. E. Lammers and A. Verhey (Grand Rapids, MI: William B. Eerdmans, 1987) and Arthur Kleinman, *The Illness Narratives: Suffering, Healing, and the Human Condition* (New York: Basic Books, 1988).

12. Toombs (this volume) writes powerfully about this dual relationship of self to body. So too does Lysaught (this volume). See also Elaine Scarry, *The Body in Pain: The Making and Unmaking of the World* (New York: Oxford University Press, 1985) and Kleinman, *Illness Narratives.*

13. Susan Brison, *Aftermath: Violence and the Remaking of a Self* (Princeton, NJ: Princeton University Press, 2002), 44.14. Ibid., 31, 44. For discussion of the limits of our capacity to regulate and control emotional states, see Care, "Problematic Agency," Judith Herman, *Trauma and Recovery: The Aftermath of Violence—*

From Domestic Abuse to Political Terror (New York: Basic Books, 1997), and Daniel J. Siegel, *The Developing Mind: How Relationships and the Brain Interact to Shape Who We Are* (New York: Guildford Press, 1999).

15. Brison, *Aftermath*, 39–40. Also see Herman, *Trauma and Recovery*, esp. chapters 2 and 3.

16. Brison, *Aftermath*, 59.

17. Edmund Pellegrino and D. C. Thomasma, *A Philosophical Basis of Medical Practice: Toward a Philosophy and Ethic of the Healing Professions* (New York: Oxford University Press, 1981), 207. See also Pellegrino and Thomasma, *For the Patient's Good* (New York: Oxford University Press, 1988).18. Warren Reich offers a beautiful discussion of suffering, which he distinguishes from "pain." Reich, "Speaking of Suffering: A Moral Account of Compassion," *Soundings* 72, no. 1 (1989): esp. 85–86.

19. For eloquent and frank discussion of this, see Scarry, *Body in Pain*.

20. In literature on suffering and trauma, an oft-repeated theme is that of having "died," or having lost one's former self. So too is the experience of isolation and alienation. See Herman, *Trauma and Recovery*, Brison, *Aftermath*, and Primo Levi, *Survival in Auschwitz* (New York: Simon and Schuster, 1958).

21. Dorothee Soelle, *Suffering*, trans. E. R. Kalin (Philadelphia: Fortress, 1975), 69. Also see Scarry, *Body in Pain*, 13, for analysis of the "inexpressibility" of pain, its "assault on language." "Pain," Scarry writes, "does not simply resist language but actively destroys it, bringing about an immediate reversion to a state anterior to language, to the sounds and cries a human being makes before language is learned." Ibid., 4; see also, more generally, 3–19. Also see Reich, *Speaking of Suffering*, who offers a compelling account of the loss of language in suffering.

22. Robert Stolorow, "Worlds of Trauma," in *Worlds of Experience: Interweaving Philosophical and Clinical Dimensions in Psychoanalysis*, by Robert Stolorow, George Atwood, and Donna M. Orange (New York: Basic Books, 2002), 124.

23. Ibid., 128; Herman, *Trauma and Recovery*, esp. chapter 3, offers a close study of social "disconnection" in the wake of traumatic experience.

24. Simone Weil, *Gravity and Grace*, trans. A. Wills (Lincoln: University of Nebraska Press, 1952), 48.

25. Brison attests to the tendency on the part of assault victims to blame themselves both to avoid "feeling overwhelmed by helplessness" and to retain a sense of "control." *Aftermath*, 74.

26. In examining cases in which the body is "invaded, injured, defiled," in contexts of rape and warfare combat, Herman writes: "Shame is a response to helplessness, the violation of bodily integrity, and the indignity suffered in the eyes of another person." *Trauma and Recovery*, 53.

27. I take this expression from Sandra Bartky, *Femininity and Domination* (New York: Routledge, 1990).

28. MacIntyre, *Dependent Rational Animals*, 2, 73.

29. Not all forms of dependency and felt need are, of course, legitimate or morally healthy.

30. Jodi Halpern, *From Detached Concern to Empathy* (New York: Oxford University Press, 2001), 85. Here I draw from Alisa Carse, "The Moral Contours of Empathy," *Ethical Theory and Moral Practice* 8 (2005): 169–95.

31. Halpern, *From Detached Concern to Empathy*, 84–85.

32. Adrian Piper, "Impartiality, Compassion, and Model Imagination," *Ethics* 101, no. 4 (1991): 726–59.

33. Halpern, *From Detached Concern to Empathy*, 33.

34. Ibid., 130.

35. Nel Noddings, *Caring: A Feminine Approach to Ethics and Moral Education* (Berkeley: University of California Press, 1984), 24.

36. Ibid., 30.

37. Of course, in the case of some conditions (e.g., sudden, strenuously debilitating diseases or injuries), "integration" may be close to impossible. In such cases, others' compassionate presence can in and of itself be meaningful.

38. Lawrence Blum, "Particularity and Responsiveness," in *The Emergence of Morality in Young Children*, ed. J. Kagan and S. Lamb (Chicago: Chicago University Press, 1989), 313.

39. Here I follow quite closely Herman's characterization of "a healing relationship." *Trauma and Recovery*, chapter 7, esp. 134. Halpern, *From Detached Concern to Empathy*, offers a compelling analysis of the role of empathy in facilitating agency, which I address later.

40. "Vicarious possession" is Adrian Pipers vivid term, referring to a problematic mode of engagement in which "one empathically experiences the other's feelings as one imagines them *to the exclusion of one's own reactions to them*." Piper, "Impartiality, Compassion, and Model Imagination," 740 (emphasis mine). Let me emphasize that being empathic does not require accepting the verity of the other's perception. Nor does it require yielding to the other's desires or expectations, for they might be unrealistic. Instead, it entails an ability to deftly distance ourselves from the other's perspective when this is needed, even while apprehending and sustaining a felt connection with his or her state. For a beautiful discussion of this challenge, see Ethel Person, *Dreams of Love and Fateful Encounters: The Power of Romantic Passion* (New York: Penguin, 1988), esp. 137–61. I explore this issue in detail in Carse, "Moral Contours of Empathy."

41. Halpern makes the point that what she calls emotional "contagion" can go both ways. For example, a physician can be infected by "a patient's catastrophic thinking," and physicians can also convey their anxieties to their patients, who "catch" the physician's fear. *From Detached Concern to Empathy*, , 10.

42. See Carse, "Moral Contours of Empathy," for more extensive exploration of the perils of limited imagination.

43. See Reich, *Speaking of Suffering*, for insightful discussion of silent presence as well as of "expressive suffering," "lamentation," and the transformative power of narrative.

44. Siegel, *Developing Mind*, 69–70.

45. Stolorow, Atwood, and Orange, *Worlds of Experience*, 128.

46. Jodi Halpern, *Concretized Emotions and Deliberative Incapacity*, unpublished manuscript.

47. Ibid., 18.

48. Ibid., esp. 26–38.

49. Brison, *Aftermath*, offers an extensive, important study of the role of narrative in recovering from trauma. Soelle, *Suffering*, and Reich, *Speaking of Suffering*,

explore the significant role of narrative in emerging from the isolation of suffering more generally.

50. Brison, *Aftermath,* 54.

51. Ibid.

52. Herman, *Trauma and Recovery,* 174.

53. See Brison, *Aftermath,* esp. 21, 49–66; also Herman, *Trauma and Recovery,* chapter 9; and Scarry, *Body in Pain,* esp. chapter 3.54. Blum, "Particularity and Responsiveness," 720–21.

55. The compounding of vulnerabilities is dramatically apparent in health care contexts, particularly in the care of patients or the treatment of research subjects. Relationships with patients and "subjects" are characterized by clear disparities of knowledge, need, and power and thus introduce a broad array of vulnerabilities; the welfare and dignity of those most dependent and needful is profoundly subject to the quality of care they receive. See Pellegrino and Thomasma, *Philosophical Basis of Medical Practices* and *For the Patient's Good.*

56. I am grateful to participants of the Theological Anthropology for Bioethics Conference for urging me to include discussion of the crucial role of solidarity in human flourishing, an insight central to the Catholic common good tradition.

57. MacIntyre, *Dependent Rational Animals,* 130.

58. Here, in the Aristotelian sense, clearly intended by MacIntyre.

59. There are, of course, already professions and enterprises oriented around compassion and solidarity—e.g., the "healing" professions, relief organizations, and many nongovernmental organizations (NGOs). I am suggesting the need for a general cultural shift.

60. MacIntyre highlights what he refers to as "the virtues of acknowledged dependency" (119), including "the attentive and affectionate regard of others." *Dependent Rational Animals,* 120–22.

61. See Cahill, this volume, for a discussion of actual, ongoing work grounded in the Catholic common good tradition and embodying a social ethic that gives a central place to human solidarity.

3

Pluralism, Truthfulness, and the Patience of Being

William Desmond

"Truth exists. Only lies are invented."

—George Braques

Truth and Construction

How we understand truth cannot be disconnected from how we understand ourselves or from how we understand how we humans are to be. "How we are to be" indicates the human being as a creature with a certain *promise of being* that calls out to be realized in one way or other. Some ways will enable fulfillment of the promise if we are true to what we are. Some ways may betray the promise if we are false to what we are. The intimate connection of being human and being true is not a merely theoretical issue but has inescapable ethical and indeed religious significance.

In philosophy we are familiar with a plurality of significant theories of truth. I will mention a few of them. There is the correspondence theory: Truth is the correlation, more or less exact, of our intellect to things. There is the coherence theory: What is most important is not an external correspondence but the immanent self-consistency of our concepts or thoughts or propositions. There are idealistic theories in which the identity of being and thought is claimed, or in which, in Hegel's famous words, "the true is the whole." There are pragmatic theories of truth: Truth is what works for us, in the long run. And there are more.

This plethora of theories might seem congenial to the contemporary ethos, which seems highly pluralistic. Yet none of these theories celebrates sheer plurality in an undiscriminating way. Our diverse answers to the question of truth call us back from any attitude that endorses "anything goes." Not everything goes. There are different senses of being true, some more appropriate to more objective determinations of actuality, some more fitting for the elusive enigmas of the human heart. To be true to something is to enact a certain fidelity to that thing, hence, depending on that thing, our "being true" will be different. There is a pluralism with regard to "being true" in that sense, but this does not preclude something more than mere plurality. I will come to this later in terms of the spirit of truthfulness.[1]

Nevertheless, in the contemporary pluralistic ethos, I do think there is a fairly widespread attitude that is worth noting, which is the view that connects *the true* and *the constructed*. Truth is our construction. Initially, one might think this is a fine view. Not only do we, the constructors of truth, become the sources of truth, but we also become its masters. What better augury for the betterment of the human condition and the pathway toward the (true) self-empowerment of man? Of course, the practices of science and medicine are one central area where this self-empowerment is at issue. If we are such constructors, perhaps we can reconstruct the conditions of life that will overcome the given patiences that often drag down our energies, such as sickness, disease, death, everything bearing on our frail, finite bodies. Truth as a construction seems to offer a marvelous beacon of hope.

There is a widespread cultural attitude that endorses a pluralism of approaches to things, a pluralism possibly unlimited, except perhaps by the powers of human invention and imagination. The call: celebrate the many, let a thousand flowers bloom. This is not unconnected with a democratic ethos in which each person is said to deserve the same respect as the next person. It is not unconnected with a view of tradition as a hegemonic univocalism, which subordinates differences to a tyrannical homogeneity. Truth, with a capital T, is judged guilty of such a tyranny. We must not seek Truth, but truths, or as Nietzsche claimed, my truth. Let a thousand truths bloom. But this is entirely too passive: let us *make* a thousand truths.

Again, in this view, everything tends to revolve around the power of creativity or the force of free imagination. In Nietzsche's writings, the poet or the artist generally enjoys a preeminence: they are the creators par excellence and, hence, in a sense dictate the truth that is to be. There is no truth that is; truth is to be what we determine it to be, and in terms of certain values we consider the most important for life. (I only mention in passing that there is often a half-hidden metaphysical presupposition, which is that reality in itself has a dark, ugly side: art saves us from this truth; art gives us the constructed truth that allows us to live.)

The true is the made, so said Vico. *Verum et factum convertuntur.* The human being can only know what it makes: hence human truths are appropriate to us. God makes the world, and hence can know it. We can know what is proportionate to us. Marx liked to quote Vico's maxim, but making for Marx becomes unanchored from the idea that there is a creator other than the human being. The human being is the only creator in a godless world. As the creators, the workers and makers of this world, we become the truth of this world, and indeed, through our own work, the creators of value also. The difference between Marx and Nietzsche is not so much on this score—it is more an accent than a basic metaphysical difference—will to power as industrial production, will to power as poetic creativity.

Although Marx is now in retreat, the attitudes he expresses are not quite so. We see this with Nietzsche, the patron saint of postmodern pluralism. And perhaps it is not surprising that the pluralism of the postmodern ethos throws us that strange mutant: the left-wing Nietzschean. Truth is what we construct, but to construct we also have to destroy, which means that we have to transgress what is traditionally taken to be truth. Assault on the old truth is part of the intoxication of constructing the new truth. Once again, it seems that we must overcome the inhibition of the (moral) imagination to unleash hitherto untapped sources of creativity and construction in ourselves.

Between Absolute Truth and Truthfulness

I rehearse a widespread view that I do not endorse. One need not deny a certain qualified creativity to the human being, but the meaning of the qualification is all-important.

The pluralism of truths often goes with, as I said, a perception of traditional theories of truth, especially the correspondence theory, as hegemonic and totalitarian. The truth, the absolute truth, is just there and given, and to it we must submit; and then, the complaint goes forth, the putative possessors of the absolute truth are repressing us.

An interesting issue is presented here. Perhaps we do not possess the absolute truth. Perhaps only God can and does. That we do not possess the absolute truth is not a postmodern view—it is as old as Plato. Human beings are not God, hence we do not—and in a sense cannot—possess the absolute truth. But the consequence does not follow that we are simply to construct what truths we consider relevant or interesting for ourselves. We do not possess absolute truth, yet we seek the truth or the true. And we could not seek at all were there not some relation between us, our desire, and the truth sought. To seek is always to be related to the truth sought. Hence, to know that we do not have the absolute truth is already to be in relation to truth. Otherwise, we could not know our ignorance nor seek what we lack and obscurely anticipate. In short, we are intermediate beings: neither in absolute possession of truth nor in absolute destitution, but somewhere in between.

The important point is that this condition is not something we construct. The "somewhere between" is the space, indeed the ethos of being, within which we might seek to construct, but it is presupposed by all our constructing power. Our being in the *metaxu* (Greek for "between") defines our participation in the milieu of being within which our own middle being intermediates with the truth—truth that might well be beyond us, though not out of relation to us. In other words, there is a relation to the truth that is prior to, and more ultimate than, any claim made that the truth is something we construct. We are in the space of truth, or truthfulness, which itself contributes to our own endowment with capacities to discern the difference between truth and falsehood, and more mediately, this truth and that. To have that endowment is to be marked by something given, not something we construct through ourselves alone. Gift is prior to construction.

You might still wonder about significance. I think it immediately calls forth a different relation to the whole question of truth. It makes us understand ourselves differently, including the fragility of our finite being, and not least how we relate to our incarnate condition. It evokes a respect, indeed reverence, for something that we do not ourselves create or construct, but that is intimately necessary for the truthfulness and worthiness of all our own efforts at constructive or creative life. There is a call of truth on us that is coeval with our being: It is constitutive of the kinds of beings we are. It releases us into a certain freedom of seeking, but this freedom and release are not themselves self-produced. There is something more at work in our searches for truth than simply our own searching and the results of that searching.

Truth and Truthfulness: Our Intermediate Being

If we take seriously the intermediate nature of the human being, what becomes evident is quite opposite to an "anything goes" attitude to truth. Rather, there emerges in our very searching a call to fidelity to truth we do not possess, and yet that endows us with something eminently distinctive. It is somewhat paradoxical that the constructivist view (as we might call it) emerges from a deep *skepticism* about truth: the traditional view that we can know the truth in itself is questioned, and indeed despaired of. And there is a switch from a sense of truth as other to us to a sense of ourselves as capable of making what truths we need in the circumstances we find ourselves. Here is the paradox: We veer from a skepticism that is stymied by the difficulty of such an ideal of truth to an orientation in which "truth" seems far more easily to hand, in what we construct ourselves. And since this last seems to be within our power, instead of skepticism about the otherness of truth, we can be given over to intoxication with our own truth-making capacities. We reject the god of absolute truth, but there is a new god in the wings, and mirabile dictu, this god is we ourselves. We are finally now liberated as self-liberating, autonomous creators.

I see our intermediate being differently. Let us grant that we do not possess absolute truth. Then this very granting is itself witness to our participation in truth *not constructed*. To say "granted" is to give oneself over to something we do not construct ourselves: We grant that something had to be accepted as granted. It is true that we do not possess the absolute truth, and so we are in intimate relation to truth, no matter that we do not know the absolute truth. We are constrained by a necessity that limits all our pretensions to absoluteness, as well as all claims to unconstrained constructivism.

The point could be put less negatively. It is not just a matter of showing certain deep instabilities in denying a sense of truth that is not our own construction, although this is important. Rather, it is a matter of attending to the fact that in the search for all truth, even in the denial that we possess the truth, we are called upon to "be truthful." One can be truthful, even in searching for the truth and even in knowing that one does not possess the truth. Our being truthful is testament to the intermediate condition of the

human seeker as between the fullness of truth of the divine and the ignorance of the beast: beyond the second, though the first be beyond us, and
yet in intimate relation to what is so beyond us, by virtue of the call to be
truthful.

Being truthful is an exigence that makes a call on us before we endeavor
to construct any system of science or philosophy that might claim to be
true. It may call us actively to construct, but the call itself shows us to be
open to something other than our own self-determination, something that
endows us with a destiny to be truthful to the utmost extent of our human
powers. In that regard, there is no way of separating the theoretical and the
practical, the metaphysical and the ethical. Being truthful is also called to
a fidelity that solicits a way of life appropriate to it, that issues in a way of
being mindful in which we are to live truthfully, and to live truly.

Being truthful is not an objective truth that lies out there somewhere,
univocally fixed in advance. It has more to do with the immanent porosity
of the human being to being as it is, and to what is good and worthy in itself
to be affirmed. It may be the case that there are forms of truth that take
on a more objective and univocal character such as we find in the so-called
hard sciences. I think this is true. But the search for such truths testifies to
another sense of being truthful, which is as much an ethical as a theoretical
demand. For instance, the scientist seeking objective truth must be faithful
to the call of being truthful—else the whole edifice of objective science is
itself corrupted. Once again, it is a sense of truthfulness having to do with
what we are: not what we seek simply, not what we are simply, but what we
are to be, as beings that seek truth and that seek to be truthful.

And yet, if it is not simply objective, it is not simply subjective, either.
We know the call to be truthful intimately in our own selves, but there is
something transsubjective about it. Something here comes to us, something
here endows us, something here gifts us with a power we could not produce
through ourselves alone. The spirit of truthfulness in us points to something transsubjective in our own selves or subjectivity. As transsubjective,
it is "objective" in the sense that it is other to us, even as it is in intimate
relation to us. But it is not objective in terms of this object or that. In that
regard, the spirit of truthfulness witnesses in what is objective to something
that is transobjective. Without it we would have no participation in objective truth, but it is not this or that objective truth, but our participation in
something more fundamental.

I might put it in terms of Pascal's very helpful distinction between *l'esprit
de géométrie* and *l'esprit de finesse.* The former is appropriate to objective

truths, such as that which we pursue in the hard sciences and mathematics. But the latter is required when we deal with the human being, in the deep ambiguity of its being, somewhere between nothing and infinity, marked alike by wretchedness and glory and called into relation to God, beyond all our knowing had not God already mysteriously made himself known to us. The spirit of truthfulness, our being truthful, is first more related to *l'esprit de finesse* than to *l'esprit de géométrie*, which is not to say that the latter does not participate in it. In a sense, this spirit of truthfulness transcends the difference of the two, if we are tempted to see them as dualistically opposed. But it is itself intimate to the finesse of the human being.

Finesse is very important in a time such as ours in which *l'esprit de géométrie* is often in the ascendant.[2] Finesse is more a readiness for a more intimate knowing, with a bearing on what is prior to and beyond geometry. It bears on a mindfulness that can read the signs of the equivocality of human existence, and not simply by the conversion of these signs into a univocal science or a philosophical system. In a way, here the power of the poetic come into its own, as well as its sister, religious reverence. Finesse is by its nature an excellence of mindfulness that is singularly embodied. It cannot be rendered without remainder in terms of neutral and general characteristics. It cannot be geometricized. We come first to know of it, know it, by witnessing its exemplary incarnation in living human beings of evident finesse. There is no geometrical "theory" that could render it in an absolutely precise univocal definition.

Finesse refers us to the concrete suppleness of living intelligence that is open, attentive, mindful, and attuned to the occasion in all its elusiveness and subtlety. We take our first steps in finesse by a kind of creative mimesis, by trying to liken ourselves to those who exemplify it or show something of it. This creative likening renews the promise of finesse, but it also is itself new because it is an openness to the subtlety of the occasion in its unrepeatable singularity. Singularity here does not betoken a kind of autism of being, nor does it mean that any communication of its significance to others is impossible. Rather, this singularity is rich with a promise, perhaps initially not fully communicated, and yet making itself available for communicability. Communicability itself cannot be confined to articulation in neutral generality or homogeneous universality. Finesse is in attendance on what is elusive in the intimacy of being, but that intimacy is at the heart of living communicability.

Consider the dominance of the often scientific and cybernetic forms of thinking in our time. These are often complemented by a kind of self-serving subjectivity in which the gratification of private desires is the point of it all. Think of the paradox of how the Internet—extraordinary result of cybernetic thinking and *l'esprit de géométrie*—is infested with pornographic sites. On the one hand, hard geometrical heads and, on the other, the mush of erotic exploitation without the heart of reverence and modesty.

Pascal's sense of finesse is very appropriate to postmodern pluralism, which often claims to celebrate amibiguity, equivocity, and so on. But finesse has to do with a discernment of what is worthy to be affirmed in the ambiguity. It is not the indiscriminate glorification of ambiguity. It is the excellence of mindfulness that does not deny the ambiguity, is not false to it, but seeks to be true to what is worthy to be affirmed in it—and not everything is worthy to be affirmed. If nothing else, finesse is not a matter of construction. Quite the opposite, the gifts that it fosters are receptivity; attention; mindfulness of singular occasions, happenings, and persons; openness to the singularity of things; readiness for the surprising and the genuine other—a feeling for the intimacy of being itself and intimate nourishment of the spirit of truthfulness in our own selves. Religion and art have been the great mistresses of finesse in the past. Without finesse, in circumstances of ethical ambiguity, there is no discerning ethical judgment. Without finesse, there is no serious and profound philosophy. Without finesse in politics, the huckster or worse usurps the place of the statesman.

Truthfulness and the Patience of Being

Finesse, and not just geometry alone, is needful in the practice of medicine. But we live in a time of ascendant geometry, and it is not always clear if we have the finesse to match what geometry constructs. I now want to connect more explicitly these remarks on truthfulness with anthropological consequences that have an ethical and theological bearing. I connect this bearing with the patience of being.

I mean that the constructivist generally thinks that our being is to do, to act: in the beginning and in the end, and in the middle is the act, the constructive act. My point is not a denial of construction but a relativization of any tendency to absolutize its claims. Our constructive act is not the first or the last or the middle. This follows from the sense of being truthful outlined earlier. The spirit of being truthful indicates first on our part a certain patience to the truth before we are called to be truthful in a more active sense. We find ourselves in the middle space between absolute ignorance and absolute truth. We do not create this middle space; it is wherein the spirit of being truthful makes its solicitation to us. We need finesse to be attentive about this because it is not merely an objective truth nor merely a subjective opinion or preference, though it is intimate to us, hence subjective, and yet other to subjectivity, hence objective in the sense of being other than our construction—it is not "made up."

I would say that there is a patience of being before there is an endeavor to be, a receiving of being before an acting of being, in accord with our singular characters as humans. The patience and receiving make the endeavor and the acting possible, and when acknowledged with finesse, patience and receiving are understood differently than from within a philosophy that wants the self-absolutizing of our activist character, or our endeavor to be.

There is a *passio essendi* more primal than the *conatus essendi*. Spinoza used this last phrase to describe the essence of a being: the essence of a being is its *conatus*—and this is defined by its power to affirm itself and its range. This range for Spinoza is potentially unlimited in the absence of external countervailing beings who express their power of being in opposition to us, or in limitation. *Conatus* is the being of a being; it is the being of the human being. Without an external limitation, the endeavor to be is potentially infinite, like a motion that will continue indefinitely without a check from the outside. One might infer from this, in the sphere of human relations, that an external other always presents itself as potentially hostile to my self-affirming. The other, so seen, while needful for my flourishing, is potentially alien to my self-affirmation, and hence one strategy of continuing the *conatus* will be for one to disarm that other in advance. Big fish, eating little fish, grow bigger.

Such a relation of implicit hostility can define our embodied relation to the rest of nature. The latter as other can be as much the source of our sustenance as a threat to the integrity of our healthy self-affirming being. It is equivocal, but the equivocal face is most known in the threat to us—in disease, infection, and finally death. Against this equivocality, we must protect ourselves by overcoming the threat. By contrast, in this view a passivity is something to be avoided or overcome. Being patient to something places us in a position of subordination—to receive from the other is taken as a sign of weakness. To receive is to be servile, whereas to act and to endeavor is to be sovereign. The emotions, for instance, are servile; the dominating reason is sovereign. One sees how this fits in with the ethos of modernity in which the autonomous subject as self-law is implicitly in ambiguous, potentially hostile relation to what is other, or *heteros*.

Some of these concerns seem to me to be in the background of the constructivist theory of truth. We are not gifted with truth, or even with the power to discern truth as other to us, but we make it for ourselves: For we ourselves are the truth of the construction. We self-construct—even to the point of constructing and reconstructing the bodies originally given to us, or of which we are originally the victims, because we did not first choose our bodies.

What of the *passio essendi*? We are first given to be, before anything else. At a theological level this bears on our being creations. Creatures of an absolute source that gives us to be and gives us to be as good: This is the good of the "to be" in which we participate but that we do not construct—but rather that allows us to construct.

The view here goes at a different angle to the modern constructivist view, but it is dependent on the recognition of an otherness more original than our own self-definition. We are only self-defining because we have originally been given to be as selves, and as selving; only creative because created; only courageous because encouraged; only loving because already loved and shown to be worthy of love; only become good to the degree that we are grateful for a good we do not ourselves produce; only become truthful because there is a truth more original than ourselves that endows us with the power to seek truth and the confidence that, should we search truly, we will find that truth (insofar as this can be understood by the finite human being).

Being patient, or being in the patience of being, is not here a defect. It is only a defect from the point of view of a *conatus* given over to the temptation to affirm itself alone, and hence closed off from the acknowledgment that it is at all because it is first affirmed to be: created.[3]

What I am saying is no denial of the *conatus*, but rather a changed vision of it that sees it as deriving from something other than itself. If we think of *the healthy body*, we immediately see something of the *conatus* in the will to self-perpetuation and self-affirmation that marks it. This is our being—to affirm itself, and indeed to affirm itself as good—it is good to be. I do not deny this at all. The question is its meaning and whether there is something more that relativizes self-affirmation—gives it to be at all and makes it porous relative to something other than itself, and not just as a servile passivity. In fact, we find ourselves in this self-affirmation; we do not first construct it. Spontaneously, we live this affirmation of the "to be" as good—we do not first have a choice—it is what we are. And since we find ourselves as thus self-affirming, there is a patience to this primal self-affirmation. Again there is something received in our being given to be, something not constructed through our own powers alone.

Of course, we have to say "yes" to this original "yes" to being, and we can develop our powers diversely. The endeavor to be in a more self-chosen way here emerges, and necessarily so. If we decide to live in a healthy way, it is following on the first "yes," but it is the living of a second "yes" that tries to respect, for instance, the integrity of the body, to live with finesse for its subtle rhythms, to embody a kind of reverence, even for a sort of sanctity that is intimate to the human body. But none of this tells against the more primal patience.

Modern constructivism forgets or wants to forget this patience. There is even a hatred of that patience that can come to be expressed, for all patience is a reminder of our status as finite creatures, and hence is a constitutive sign of the fact that we are not the masters of being, not even of our own being. The weaknesses of the latter are often rejected, refused. And there is a qualified sense in which that refusal has some right. But when it loses any porosity to the more primal patience, its seeming self-affirmation is really a kind of self-hatred, for this endeavor to be is in flight from itself, from what it is, from the patience of being that gives it to be at all in the first instance. The conditions that make possible its being at all are refused. Hence, we find ourselves in the impossible situation of the flower trying to ingest its own ground—impossible, yet were it even conceivable, it would show the inner self-hatred of the flower that must only destroy itself in this way of absolutizing itself.

One wonders about how much of modern constructivism is in flight from this patience, and hence from itself, even when it seems to flee only to itself. The patience of being shows what is not our own, even in what is most intimately our own. Just so, the spirit of being truthful shows some sense of truth more primally other than our self-determination, in the deepest intimacy of our own self-determination.

Being Truthful and Patience

Being truthful is impossible without this patience. It calls for the practice of finesse: This is a matter of giving the time for this patience in order to attend to what is both within us and before us. True, given the energies that carry our endeavor to be, it tends to happen again and again that there is an *overriding* of this patience by the *conatus*. Being alive is to find oneself always tempted to this impatient overriding. The fulfillment of life is impossible if this happens. We have not taken the proper time nor respected the rhythms of time to attend to what is within us and before us, and hence to be truthful concerning our proper response to the promise of our being, and indeed to its sickness, when we have deserted what is good in promising. This is also to say that the very healthy perpetuation of life is conditional on a perpetual recurrence of the patience, and a perpetual receiving of the promise of life. This recurrence and this receiving come to their term when we meet the limit of mortality: When death reveals the finitude that calls time on the endeavor to be.

This recurrence of patience, however, is not only a matter of when the endeavor to be meets an external or hostile limit and is brought low. It is always happening, and its gift of promise is always being offered, even though we do not notice or acknowledge it. It concerns the gift of life as received, granted to us in the first instance, but in the rush forward of the endeavor to be, taken for granted rather than as granted. In the sweep of a life, the external limits of encroaching others, or the limit of mortal time, both internal and external, can serve as reminders of this more primal patience of being, in which we may again consent to the goodness of the gift of life. Alternatively, at the other extreme, we may continue to turn against its givenness in rejection just because it is given and not produced by us: not made by us, hence beyond our full self-determination. We can insist that everything be subject to our self-determination that we betray the joy of this gift in the overriding of our own self-affirmation. Consent to death, in gratitude for the gift of life, is our final opportunity to make our peace with this patience.

Being Patient and Being Incarnate

This patience of being is intimately related to our incarnate being. Being incarnate is first something given before we "construct" it as other than given. We do the latter, for instance, in adornment, or in interventions that strengthen the body, such as athletic training, or in medical interventions that normally are for purposes of allowing the body as it is to regain itself and its native energies. Initially we are patient with these energies of the body, though these energies are themselves active and dynamic—and most especially when we are young. They live us instead of us always directing them. It is entirely fitting that we come to direct them as best we can, and in the light of what we discern to be the best for ourselves. But we are not always wise in our directions, and again more likely unwise than wise if we forget this patience of being and override its more finessed insinuations with a too self-insistent endeavor to be. Even when the energies of the body are brought toward their maximal expression, there is needed a kind of fidelity to this patience—it is not a matter of just exerting oneself, though it is obviously this, too. There is more than self-exertion when this maximum is approached.

Thus, athletes will speak of remaining relaxed even while still striving, or of finding oneself in the zone, or of being in the flow, and then one is flowing—as if asleep in one sense, but awakened in an intense awareness that takes no notice of itself. I think of the Buddhist view: Form is emptiness, emptiness is form. I take this to mean that more often than not we get in the way of ourselves, as it were; we let the *conatus essendi* unfittingly override the *passio essendi*. And to let the flow pass, or begin to pass again, we must get out of our own way, and then we are more truly on the way, and on the way as more truly ourselves. Form is the harmony of energies working in intense accord, but the harmony must be empty of the clogging self-insistences that hinder rather than release the energies of selving. Hinder just by insisting on themselves, without patience for selving, and the other secret sources of enabling that hiddenly contribute to every act of accomplished excellence.

This asks of us also an orientation of respect and reverence for the body. Respect and reverence are family relations to patience. Each requires a mentality or mindfulness other than one that is objectifying of the body and its practical correlate, the utilitarian exploitation of the body—whether in pornographic sex, or the sale of body parts, or whatever. One might say that the patient body, understood in terms of what I discussed earlier, is already an incarnate sign of a love beyond instrumentalizing.

One might see the great artist as serving the celebration of this passion of being. One might also see those involved in the care of the sick as called to behold the bodies of the patients as incarnate signs of this love beyond instrumentalizing. The least of these are incarnate signs of the divine, calling those still in robust health to the practice of a love that also signals something beyond the instrumentalizing of the others. The service of the medical healer has always been a sign of this care beyond instrumentalizing.

In the case of human beings, this care is noteworthy in the manner it takes on certain unconditional characteristics: those who, from a biological point of view, seem worthless are deemed worthy of a sacred respect. I know there are those who will bridle at a phrase like "sacred respect." And it is only too true that there are massive trends in our time geared to the project of, so to say, *deconsecrating the human body*. The space between deconsecration and desecration is often, alas, infinitesimal. I think that the loss of the patience of being in modern Western culture is potentially disastrous: loss of the finesse needed to discern the rightness of this deeming of sacred worth. The profit and the loss of human lives are reckoned on a utilitarian calculus—to the profitless loss of being truthful to what we more intimately are.

The Patience of Being, Health, and Sickness

To be human is to be patient, but to be patient is not necessarily to be sick. It turns out also that the doctor or nurse or healer or caregiver is patient, and not only the sick person. There is a health in patience that makes possible the healing of the sick. Thus, in the relation of doctor and patient, there is the call of this patience that extends to both sides. Being truthful to the relation asks patience as much from the healthy as from the sick. Needless to say, this is often difficult, if differently difficult, on both sides: on the side of the weak because the *conatus* is laid low or enfeebled, and on the side of the still healthy because of the zest of the *conatus* and because the weak are hindrances to the blithe continuation of life. Being truthful to the more original patience can be deeply salutary in reminding us that every human being is on *both sides of this* relation; now more on this side perhaps, but in turn the reverse will be the case, and the strong will *sere*.

Yet, whether on one side or the other, or on both, there is again a deeper sense of patience that is not a matter of sickness but of mindful porosity to what transcends us. In any case, we are never just dealing with a problem to be solved by a neutral geometry, the brilliant interventions of amazing technologies, for instance. Porosity to what transcends us makes us potentially liable to attack from hostile others, human or nonhuman, but it also constitutes the promise of our community beyond hostility with others. The being truthful of finesse is always needed. And again, whether on one side or the other, or on both, this is not just a matter of judging how things stand with our own endeavor to be; it is a matter of a fidelity to the patience of our own being and that of the suffering others. One might perhaps here speak of a kind of *compassio essendi*, a compassion of being, in which both strong and weak can participate. And perhaps this *compassio essendi* communicates a sign of what a more divine love might be for mortal creatures.

The Patience of Being and Religious Porosity

One might say that perhaps the most ultimate and elusive form of finesse deals with how the patience of being brings us to the boundary of the religious. It places us in a space of porosity between the human and the divine. There we are sometimes involuntarily placed, when in sickness our helplessness is brought home to us. We might ask, "Why me?" but to whom is our defiance or appeal addressed, if there is nothing, no divine other porous to our outcry? The outcry is not just addressed to ourselves, or to human others. Either to nothing, or to God.

Those who are healthy and who wish to heal are themselves often placed in this porous space of helplessness—when they can do nothing further for the person slipping away. They too can be visited by a despair that may be a portal to religious consent—or defiance that closes down the porosity to the divine. Nevertheless, one might say that we can come to know intimately that there is a patience that is graced.

There is the harder consent of those who must say "yes" to their finitude. None of us is exempt, and we will all come to the challenge of this harder consent. In a certain regard, we are always coming to this consent, or fleeing it, in every moment of our life. There is also a graced patience in that attendance on others, which is a service of their good, even if it does little or nothing to serve the advancement of some agenda of the servant. We become witnesses to the *compassio essendi* in the care we take of the other for the sake of the other. In this care, we may be released beyond ourselves in a minding of the other potentially agapeic. One sees a certain confluence here between truthfulness and the patience of being, in love of the pluralism of creation, most known in our love of singular human beings who have been our companions on a way of mystery. Being truthful is a patient service—service of the truth of the other, as of the good that solicits our attention to the good of the others. This patience is graced because it receives in readiness, at a boundary at the limits of our self-determination. Patience lays us open to secret sources of strengthening that make us porous to the religious intermediation with the divine.

NOTES

1. On different senses of truth and being true, see my *Being and the Between* (Albany: SUNY Press, 1995), chap. 12.

2. Finesse recalls us to modes of mindfulness in attunement with the fuller subtleties at play in human existence. One need not decry geometry, but its great helpfulness with univocal exactness is not always the most helpful, particularly when we are dealing with the equivocities of the human condition. Pascal is a great exemplar of the tremendous advances in the modern scientific univocalizing

wrought by empirical and mathematical science. Unlike Descartes and Spinoza, Pascal was not bewitched by its power or seduced into making it the one and only way to truth. Spinoza is not without his own finesse, but in his ethics *more geometrico* I can find no appropriate name for its generous acknowledgment. Quite the opposite, geometry seems to be usurping the role of finesse. Spinoza makes an astonishing statement to the effect that the human race would have lain forever in darkness were it not for the development of mathematics. "Truth would be eternally hidden (*in aeternam lateret*) from the human race had not mathematics, which does not deal with ends but with the nature and properties of figures, shown to humankind another norm of truth." *Ethics*, Part I, appendix, in Carl Gebhart, ed., *Spinoza Opera* (Heidelberg: Heidelberger Akademie der Wissenschaften, 1924), 79; see *The Chief Works of Benedict de Spinoza*, trans. R. H. M. Elwes (New York: Dover Publications, 1955), 77. If I read this right, a (quasi-)soteriological power is being claimed for mathematics. Prior to the geometrical sages of modernity, humanity seems to have been lost in the caves of night. After the new mathematics, rational salvation offers humankind the possibility of release into light, into blessedness. What release, what blessedness? If mathematics saves us from purposes and ends (*fines*), would its knowing then be a purposeless knowing in a purposeless universe? If this is proffered as an advance beyond darkness, it also seems to be an advance into a different darkness, darker in its intelligibility than the unintelligible darkness we have now supposedly left behind. I wonder if we are being offered a kind of geometrical counterfeit of saving knowing. Despite the esoteric caution, moderation, and sobriety of Spinoza, one wonders if his resort to geometry masks a version of rationality as esoteric will to power: the *conatus*, knowing the mechanical causes of nature, and becoming mindful of its own self-interest, will be better able to *serve itself*, and an increase in the power of its self-affirmation? "Rational" will to power, whether of Descartes's desire to be "master and possessor of nature" or of Spinoza's perhaps more masked form, is not quite Nietzsche's "irrational" will to power, but it is still will to power. Finesse, I would say, requires a different love, before and beyond purposeless "theory."

3. The patience of being might be theologically connected with *the givenness of creation*. Frequently we take this givenness for granted. What is, as being granted, creation, is taken for granted. Nevertheless, what is taken for granted is, in its being granted. There is a primal *passio essendi*, or ontological patience of being in the given receiving of being at all. This signals an "It is" entirely different, for instance, from Hegel's mere fact or indigent being of immediacy. This deepest ontological givenness is not the spontaneous happening of this or that, or the living participating in this or that experience, undergoing, or whatever, of life. It is a more primal ontological immediacy that things are at all: in being and not nothing. This is an ultimate immediacy in that, without it nothing finite, or nothing within finitude, could mediate its being there at all. For this *being there at all* is presupposed by all such mediations; and indeed all such mediations are made possible by it as the primal immediacy of being given to be. Before this surplus happening there is agapeic astonishment, or wonder, before there is determinate or self-determining cognition. Wonder, marvel, and reverence all reveal something of what is *good and worthy of affirmation* in the patience of being, even apart from any construction or further mediations by our own endeavor to be.

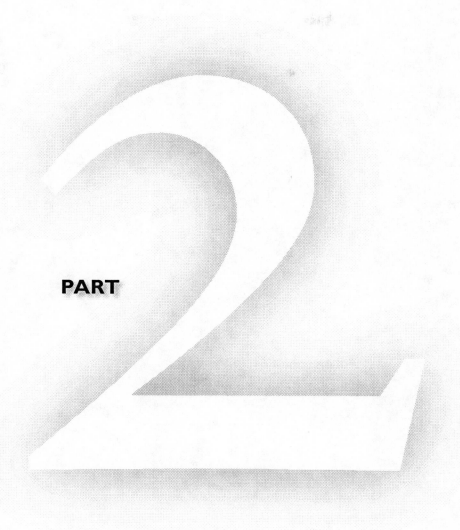

PART

2

Dignity and Integrity

4

Dignity and the Human as a Natural Kind

Daniel P. Sulmasy, O.F.M.

Dignity appears to be an important word in ethics, occurring five times in the Universal Declaration of Human Rights of the United Nations,[1] and five times in the European Convention on Human Rights and Biomedicine.[2] Ronald Dworkin has noted the fundamental moral significance of dignity, yet decried its lack of clear meaning:

> Anyone who professes to take rights seriously, and who praises our government for respecting them . . . must accept at a minimum, one or both of two important ideas. The first is the vague but powerful idea of human dignity. This idea, associated with Kant but defended by philosophers of different schools, supposes that there are ways of treating a man that are inconsistent with recognizing him as a full member of the human community, and holds that such treatment is

profoundly unjust. The second is the more familiar idea of political equality.[3]

Dworkin's complaint seems especially true in current debates about important topics in bioethics such as cloning, stem cells, and euthanasia. The word *dignity* is vague, and it is used in different ways by different speakers; therefore conceptual clarification of the word seems in order.

Elsewhere, in attempting to bring some clarity to the concept of dignity with respect to moral issues in the care of the dying, I have drawn a distinction between attributed dignity and intrinsic dignity[4] and have linked these ideas to the concept of natural kinds in an ethical analysis of euthanasia.[5] In this chapter I further refine the notions of dignity and natural kinds, noting the implications for morality of a shift from thinking about classes to kinds.

Dignity and Value Theory

Every ethical theory, implicitly or explicitly, requires a theory of value (i.e., an axiology). Classically, values have been divided into two main types—instrumental and intrinsic.[6] Instrumental values derive their significance from the purposes of the valuer. X has instrumental value to the extent that it can be used to achieve some valued outcome for P. Intrinsic value is not a function of a valuer's purposes. X has intrinsic value when it is valuable in itself.

Kant seems to place great moral emphasis on this instrumental/intrinsic difference in a way that is significantly related to his own conception of dignity: "Act in such a way that you treat humanity, whether in your own person or in the person of another, always at the same time as an end and never simply as a means."[7] Nonetheless, I hold that the relationship between value, dignity, and ethics is really much more complicated than the instrumental/intrinsic distinction.

Intrinsic Value

The field of environmental ethics has required a deep and careful exploration of the concept of intrinsic value. Laboring to understand whether species have value independent of human beings, writers such as Holmes

Rolston III have helped to clarify that there are things that have value in themselves—value that need not be conferred by a valuer. This is the value that things have by virtue of their nature and place in the universe, a value that is independent of any human evaluation. Truly intrinsic values, according to Rolston, "are objectively there—discovered, not generated by the valuer."[8] Intrinsic value is therefore more accurately defined as the value that something has solely by virtue of its intrinsic nature. No matter whether this value is recognized by external valuers, no matter whether there even *are* any external valuers, things with intrinsic value have value. The source of this value is prior to valuation.

Attributed Value: Instrumental and Noninstrumental

I call values that require a valuer *attributed values*. These values exist by virtue of the attribution of some being capable of attributing value to an individual object, natural kind, state of affairs, concept, or some other sort of thing. This is the value something has been assigned in relation to me, or to my group, or to my kind. As I noted earlier, the classical approach to value theory has been to distinguish intrinsic value from instrumental value. But this may be far too simplistic a classification.

I argue that the primary distinction in values is between the intrinsic and the attributed. There is a logical relationship between attributed values and instrumental values that may explain why it has not been noticed that the intrinsic/attributed distinction is prior to the instrumental/noninstrumental distinction. *All* instrumental values are attributed values. If they are instrumental, they are always relative to a valuer's purposes. However, not all attributed values are instrumental. For example, a watch has instrumental value in the sense that it enables me to know the time. I attribute the watch with instrumental value, and someone designed it for that purpose. But this instrumental value does not exhaust its attributed value. I may still attribute sentimental value to an old gold pocket watch that belonged to my grandfather and no longer runs and therefore has no instrumental value to me or anyone else as a timekeeping device.

Saying that something does not have instrumental value does not imply that its value is intrinsic. The mere fact that the value one attributes to an old watch is not instrumental does not necessarily imply that its value is intrinsic. The sentimental value I attach to it is not the value others would assign to it. It is not a value that is there to be discovered objectively, but a value that is attributed by a valuer. Yet its sentimental value is not instrumental. There is no outcome or purpose to my valuing this nonfunctional watch. It therefore seems that there are both instrumental and noninstrumental attributed values.

It is also important to note that attributed values can be assigned degrees. Some things will have more value in relation to the valuer than do others. Value may be attributed to a thing one day and not attributed to that same thing the next day, depending on the context and the condition of that thing. For example, an erasable marker pen has value to me when I teach in a place that has white erasable marker boards, but does not have the same value to me if I teach someplace that has only chalkboards and chalk. The attributed value of a thing can vary from valuer to valuer, or from one group of valuers to another (e.g., a culture, a nation, or the nature of the valuing entity).

Intrinsic Value and Natural Kinds

Individual entities can be said to have intrinsic value only by virtue of belonging to a natural kind.

Artifacts, by contrast with a natural kind, have only attributed value. They are, by definition, made by agents who attribute value to them, and are sometimes exchanged between agents who also attribute value to them. Generally, this attributed value is instrumental. For example, a teapot is made in order to serve the goals of its user by brewing tea and facilitating its pouring, thereby bringing about other valued states of affairs, such as keeping a professor awake while writing or expressing hospitality to a neighbor. But an artifact may also have attributed noninstrumental value. For example, an antique teapot may have aesthetic value. Such values require a valuer to attribute them to the artifact, but they are not instrumental. Further, a teapot may be used for instrumental purposes other than those intended by the maker of the teapot, such as holding and pouring soy sauce. These instrumental values can be attributed by the user on the basis of circumstance, need, or whim. But whether instrumental or noninstrumental, the value of an artifact is always attributed.

Intrinsic value is the value that something has solely by virtue of its being the kind of thing that it is. This means that the very concept of intrinsic value commits one to the concept of natural kinds.[9] If one were to propose that intrinsic value pertained to anything other than natural kinds, then the phrases "in virtue of its intrinsic nature" or "in virtue of being the kind of thing that it is" would be literally nonsense, and the concept of intrinsic value would only be confused.

If one were to reject the concept of natural kinds, one would be postulating a universe populated only by individually existing things of which properties could be predicated, arranged in various states of affairs. Things could not then be "the kinds of things that they are," but only individuals that do or do not have certain properties. If the universe really were to consist only of individuals without natural kinds, then the only thing that could truly define each individual thing "being the kind of thing that it is" would be its bare existence. But if that were true, then everything that exists would have intrinsic value in equal amounts, and one could not say that one thing had intrinsic value and another thing did not. This would render the concept of intrinsic value meaningless.

Derivative Values

Some might suggest that limiting the range of entities that have intrinsic value to members of natural kinds is too narrow a conception of intrinsic value. For example, certain processes or states of affairs are often said to have intrinsic value. However, this seems to be one of those instances in which the use of ordinary language requires some clarification and correction. The value of processes is always, by definition, instrumental, and cannot be intrinsic. The value of those states of affairs one would be inclined to call intrinsically valuable is, on reflection, derivative—dependent on the kinds of entities that are in those states of affairs.

The flourishing of a member of a natural kind is a good state of affairs, but that goodness depends on the kind of thing that is flourishing. The goodness of that state of affairs depends on some knowledge of the kind of thing that is in that state of affairs. Why a particular state of affairs is good depends on what the thing is. Thus the value of that state of affairs is derivative. One might be tempted to say that flourishing is intrinsically good, but the goodness of flourishing is always dependent on the kind of thing that is said to be flourishing, and thus that state of affairs is not, strictly speaking, intrinsically valuable.

According to this view, human virtues such as courage are not, in a technical sense, intrinsically valuable. Since the virtue of courage is a state of affairs of an individual member of the human natural kind, the value of courage is dependent on knowledge of what kind of thing a human being is. Acts that one calls courageous would not be counted as such if performed by a laboratory rat. There is no such thing as an intrinsically good disembodied Platonic Virtue. Flourishing is always the flourishing of some kind of thing. Human virtues are good because they instantiate aspects of the flourishing of the human natural kind in virtuous individuals.

Similarly, a process is not intrinsically valuable. A process is always instrumental, and its goodness depends on the outcome. If that process is conducive to the flourishing of something that is intrinsically good, one might be tempted to speak as if the process itself were intrinsically good. But again, its goodness depends on outcomes, and these in turn depend on the states of affairs of the kinds of things that constitute the outcomes. If what one means by "process" is some activity that expresses human flourishing rather than some activity that leads to human flourishing, then this sense of the word *process* refers to a state of affairs—to a virtue. But a process that leads to virtue is valued because of the virtue to which it leads. Thus no process is itself intrinsically valuable.

Yet to say that these sorts of processes and states of affairs that lead to or express human flourishing are not intrinsically valuable does not imply that the goodness of these processes and states of affairs is subjective. The value of these processes and states of affairs is not attributed by a valuer but derived from the intrinsic value of the kind under consideration. Once one knows what kind of a thing is under consideration, one can begin to specify states of affairs that instantiate its flourishing and the processes that are conducive to its flourishing as the kind of thing that it is. I will call these values *derivative values*. I suggest that there are two types of derivative value. The processes that lead to the flourishing of a natural kind I call *developmental values*, and the states of affairs that instantiate the flourishing of the kind I call *virtues*.

Natural Kinds

What is a natural kind? Although it is in many ways an ancient idea, it is a relatively new concept in analytic philosophy, designating a category of entities, all the members of which, by virtue of being brought under the extension of the kind, can be *necessarily* known to be that sort of thing. This theory argues that nature fixes certain "sortal predicates," so that it is not open to human beings to decide to classify natural kinds as anything other than what they are, for example, oxygen or a lemon or a human being.[10]

The analytical apparatus necessary to arrive at this conception is complex, but the idea, at its core, is utterly simple. What is in the world is given—in a shapely, differentiated way. There are many different *kinds* of things in the world. One has epistemic access to the kindedness of things. One can make the judgment that two individual entities, despite all their unique features, are the same kind of thing.

Logically, natural kinds are not simple classes. As Wiggins says, "[The] determination of a natural kind stands or falls with the existence of law-like principles that will collect together the actual extension of the kind around an arbitrary good specimen of it; and these law-like principles will also determine the characteristic development and typical history of members of this extension."[11]

Natural kinds thus have a natural teleology. Besides sortal predicates, they have what Lisska calls "dispositional predicates," natural tendencies to develop, behave, and flourish in certain ways as the kinds of things that they are.[12]

This is a bare-bones essentialism. As Wiggins puts it, the essences of natural kinds are not "fancied vacuities parading in the shadow of familiar things as the ultimate explanation of everything that happens in the world. They are the natures whose possession by their owners is the precondition of their owners being divided from the rest of reality as anything at all."[13] Even in a philosophical climate that is hostile to essentialism, the concept of natural kinds has made respectable again what Wiggins has called a "modest essentialism."[14]

The foregoing is not a proof that there are such things as natural kinds. I leave that to the recent cogent arguments of philosophers doing work in metaphysics.[15] However, I have explained what a natural kind is and offered an argument that if there is such a thing as intrinsic value, then it pertains to natural kinds. If one is committed to the concept of intrinsic value, one must be committed to the concept of natural kinds.

Dignity and Intrinsic Value

While all members of a particular natural kind have equal intrinsic value, the intrinsic value of different natural kinds appears to vary and admit of degrees. The intrinsic value of dirt and the intrinsic value of human beings appear to differ. There is a hierarchy of intrinsic value between and among natural kinds. However, by the definition of intrinsic value, there can be no hierarchy of intrinsic value *within* natural kinds.

I argue that the word we use to refer to the highest level of intrinsic value that a natural kind can have is *Dignity* (with a capital D). Just as there are two types of attributed value (instrumental and noninstrumental), and two types of derivative value (developmental values and virtues), so there are two types of intrinsic value (simple intrinsic value and Dignity). Dignity, in this sense of the word, is the label by which we designate those natural kinds that have certain typical characteristics that give them a particularly high intrinsic value. The kinds of dispositional predicates[16] that characterize those natural kinds that have intrinsic Dignity include the highly developed kind-typical capacities for language, rationality, love, free will, moral agency, creativity, and ability to grasp the finite and the infinite. These certainly characterize the human natural kind. But this is not to say that there might not be other natural kinds that also have such highly developed kind-typical dispositional predicates. On the supposition that angels exist, they would necessarily have intrinsic Dignity. It is quite conceivable that somewhere out there in the unimaginable immensity of the universe there might be natural kinds on other planets that have such highly developed kind-typical capacities that one would say that they also have intrinsic Dignity.

All creatures on the planet Earth have some sort of intrinsic value. In my estimation, however, none of these other natural kinds have such highly developed kind-typical capacities for language, rationality, love, free will, moral agency, creativity, aesthetic sensibility, and so on that I am willing to say that their intrinsic value reaches the threshold for calling that value Dignity. Certain sea mammals and higher primates come close, and this might merit serious discussion. But it is important to note that Dignity, as a threshold concept, pertains to a threshold among natural kinds, not individuals. Individuals have intrinsic value only by virtue of being members of a particular kind. And only the judgment that a particular natural kind is characterized by the lawlike generalizations that meet this threshold enables one to say that an individual belonging to that natural kind has intrinsic Dignity.

Only one natural kind seems sufficiently well known to us that almost everyone will agree that its members have intrinsic Dignity—the human natural kind. The argument therefore provides another way of affirming what I have elsewhere called "intrinsic human dignity."[17] This is roughly the way the word *dignity* was used by Kant when he declared that "humanity itself is a dignity"[18] and insisted that human beings be treated as ends in themselves and never purely instrumentally. Finally, it seems that this is the way the word *dignity* is used in the Universal Declaration on Human Rights and in the European Community's Convention on Human Rights and Biomedicine. This intrinsic Dignity is the value one has simply because one is a member of the human natural kind.

Noninstrumental Attributed Value: The Attributed Dignities

Unfortunately, the word *dignity* is ambiguous. Confusingly, the word *dignity* is also used to refer to attributed values. There is a very common cluster of such uses of the word *dignity*. One says, for instance, that some action is undignified or that some state of affairs has resulted in a diminution of one's dignity. Both uses refer to noninstrumental values, yet these speakers are not referring to truly intrinsic value (Dignity with a capital D). They are referring to attributed, noninstrumental values. I will use "attributed dignities" (in the plural with a small d) to refer to these attributions of nonintrinsic, noninstrumental value.

It is important to note that not all noninstrumental attributed values can be called attributed dignities (see table 4.1). Ordinary discourse further restricts the way this word is used, making it a subset of the noninstrumental attributed values. First, the word *dignity* is generally not used in attributing noninstrumental value to artifacts, but instead only to natural kinds. Bricks, for example, can have both instrumental and noninstrumental attributed value, but they have no attributed dignities. Bricks have instrumental attributed value for their use in construction. They can also have attributed noninstrumental value (e.g., aesthetic value). One might appreciate the look of a brick façade, or the surface of the bricks may be impressed with a particular design that is thought to be beautiful. These are noninstrumental attributed values. Yet bricks are not described as having "dignity." One might occasionally hear someone say that a house has "dignity," but this is generally an indirect attribution of noninstrumental value to the builder or to the interior designer or to the owner.

Second, the word *dignity* is generally used in the attributive sense only with reference to natural kinds that have intrinsic Dignity in the first place. A corn plant has both simple intrinsic value by virtue of being the kind of thing that it is, and also instrumental attributed value, by virtue of its utility as food for human beings and their livestock. But no one would say that corn has dignity, in either an attributed or an intrinsic sense.

Thus, discourse about "dignity" in the sense of the attributed dignities (with a small d) appears reserved for natural kinds that have Dignity in the intrinsic sense (with a capital D). In general, then, because we are most secure in the judgment that intrinsic Dignity belongs to human beings, the word *dignity* is reserved for discourse about human beings, even in the attributed sense.

These attributed dignities are thus a subset of noninstrumental attributed values, reserved for beings that have intrinsic Dignity (viz., human beings). In this attributed sense, one speaks, for example, of visiting "dignitaries." One claims that a certain task is "beneath one's dignity." One speaks of a person "behaving in an undignified manner." All of these, and other nonintrinsic, noninstrumental uses of the word *dignity* require a valuer—oneself or another person—to attribute the value. These uses of the word *dignity* do not refer to the value that a human being has by virtue of being a human being. That is to say, they are not referring to intrinsic values. But neither are these typically instrumental values. They do not refer to the usefulness of a human being to himself or herself or to another. These attributed dignities contribute in important ways to human flourishing. Attributed human dignities also refer to more than the preferences of individual human beings. Alongside the virtues and developmental values that derive their value from the intrinsic value (Dignity) of human beings, they help to constitute human flourishing. A complete moral theory would relate all these values to a fuller account of human excellence and flourishing, but a discussion of these issues would take us far beyond the main themes of this chapter.

As shown in table 4.1, I will consistently use the phrase "intrinsic Dignity" to refer to the special type of intrinsic value that belongs to members of those natural kinds that have kind-specific capacities for language, rationality, love, free will, moral agency, creativity, aesthetic sensibility, ability to grasp the

Table 4.1 Classification of Basic Kinds of Value

Attributed		Intrinsic		Derivative	
Instrumental values	Noninstrumental attributed values (including attributed dignities)	Simple intrinsic value	Intrinsic dignity	Developmental values	Virtues

finite and the infinite, and so on that merit this designation. I will use the phase "attributed dignities" to refer to the noninstrumental values that are attributed to members of any natural kind that has intrinsic Dignity.

Dignity: Kinds, Not Classes

Some wish to advance the claim that there can be a class of individuals within the human natural kind, none of the members of which have Dignity. Generally, they draw a distinction between members of the kind who are persons, and those who are not. For some of these commentators, the necessary and sufficient conditions for being a member of the class of persons extends beyond the human natural kind to include members of other known natural kinds, such as higher primates and certain kinds of sea mammals. Some members of the human natural kind are not, according to this view, persons, and therefore have neither Dignity nor whatever moral protections follow from having Dignity. These typically include embryonic and fetal members of the kind, those who suffer from postcoma unresponsiveness ("persistent vegetative state"), anencephalics, the severely mentally retarded, and the severely demented.

This view of personhood can certainly be debated. Boethius's classical definition of a person as "an individual substance of a rational nature"[19] can easily be translated into the language of natural kinds by saying that a person is an individual member of a natural kind that meets the threshold criteria for Dignity—rationality, freedom, capacity for grasping the finite and the infinite, morality, love, creativity, and so on. Being a member of such a kind, being a person, and having Dignity, even on this reformulation of the classical view, are coextensive and inseparable. The task of disaggregating these concepts should seem daunting to anyone who approaches the question seriously. Wiggins nicely describes what makes the disaggregation of the concepts of person and *human being* so odd and difficult even to consider when he states, "a human being is our only stereotype for *person*."[20]

But suppose one were to set aside these difficulties in order to persist boldly in the argument that only certain members of the human natural kind have Dignity. Even so, there are logical implications of such a move that raise serious questions about its validity. We have defined Dignity as an intrinsic value. Intrinsic value means the value something has by virtue of being the kind of thing that it is. Therefore those who wish to say that some members of the human natural kind do not have Dignity are left with a limited number of moves.

"Person," as the term is used in these arguments, is not a natural kind. This use of "person" denotes a class. In the standard form of this argument, the author provides a list of predicates to stipulate an intentional definition of the class. Some human beings are in the class, and some are not, depending on whether all of the necessary and sufficient characteristics of the class *person* can be predicated of them. However, it appears to have escaped much notice that if one says that Dignity comes about by meeting the necessary and sufficient conditions for being a member of a class, not by being a member of a kind, then this entails the belief that Dignity is not an intrinsic value. This follows because classes have necessary and sufficient conditions that are stipulated. Stipulation is a form of attribution. And so, if Dignity is based on membership in a class rather than a kind, Dignity would be an attributed value not an intrinsic value, contradicting our working definition of Dignity, subverting what most people mean by the word. If any value is thought to be intrinsic, it is fundamental human Dignity. And if it is truly an intrinsic value, it cannot be "up to us." Dignity commands recognition and respect. It is not up to me (or us, collectively) to decide who has Dignity and who does not—unless Dignity is not an intrinsic value.

A truly intrinsic value is not merely a name given to a class of individuals that share particular predicates. Intrinsic value, by definition, is the value that pertains to a thing by virtue of its being the kind of thing that it is. Classes of things, based solely on predicable properties, cannot constitute an intrinsic nature.

To see why this is so, consider the example of a diamond. Diamonds are valued as a natural kind because of the characteristics that are typical of the diamond as a natural kind—their hardness, brilliance, refractive capacities, and so on. Certainly much of the value of a diamond is attributed—it is conferred upon these gems by human valuers. But part of the value of a diamond is intrinsic. It depends upon an individual diamond's being the kind of thing that it is. Suppose that someone were able to manufacture a fake diamond that had all of the characteristics of a real diamond that are deemed, by attribution, worthy of admiration. Suppose further that it were manufactured in such a way as to imitate a diamond so well that even the expert appraisers at the diamond market in Amsterdam were fooled. Suppose it were later discovered that this gem were a "fake." It would still be in the class of those things that share all the valued predicates that are typical of genuine diamonds, but that would not be enough to give it the equivalent *intrinsic* value of a diamond. It would not be the kind of thing that a diamond is. In fact, a defective gem that belongs genuinely to the natural kind of diamonds is more valuable than any of the "perfect" artificial gems that are now available on the market.

One should note further that the intrinsic value of any individual member of particular natural kind is always equal to that of any other member of the same natural kind. Unlike attributed value, the intrinsic value of a thing does not admit of degrees once one knows what kind of a thing it is. The intrinsic value of a thing does not depend on its value to a valuer, how it is perceived by a valuer, or on any group of valuers. The intrinsic value of a thing would appear to be inalienable. Intrinsic value cannot be divorced from the thing itself. This is why even a thinker such as Dworkin must acknowledge that people have rights because the rest of us first recognize that they have Dignity. We do not attribute Dignity to them to the extent that we have first attributed rights to them.

As I argued earlier, intrinsic value belongs to natural kinds, not classes. The intrinsic Dignity of a demented member of the human natural kind, according to my theory, is the same as the intrinsic Dignity of a philosopher-king. The attributed dignities of the two may differ drastically. There may be a moral mandate to build up the attributed dignities of the demented patient. But arguments about whether the demented patient is a person are moot with respect to intrinsic Dignity. "Person," as it is typically used in such arguments, denotes a class. Intrinsic Dignity, like any intrinsic value, belongs to individuals by virtue of the fact that they are members of natural kinds, not classes.

The "Not Human" Counterargument

A more radical approach by those who wish to deny Dignity to certain classes of human beings would be to deny that embryos, fetuses, anencephalics, retarded infants, the demented, and permanently unresponsive adults are members of the human natural kind, that is, the argument that not only do these individuals fail to meet the criteria for personhood, but they are not human.

But this seems not so much radical as absurd. Natural kinds are not arbitrary classes created by human will. Natural kinds have a mind-to-world

84 DANIEL P. SULMASY, O.F.M.

direction of fit, that is, our understanding must be fitted to the kind; the kind is not shaped to our understanding of it.[21] Once one knows what a natural kind is, it becomes easy to recognize that the retarded, anencephalics, and the permanently unresponsive are all members of the human natural kind, albeit damaged. Zygotes, embryos, and fetuses are members of the human natural kind at the earliest stages of development. These words are for phase-sortals, not kind-sortals. These words describe phases in the development of various natural kinds, and thus make reference to the kind. A human embryo is a phase in the development of the human natural kind, and a porpoise embryo is a phase in the development of the natural kind of porpoises. Phases are not distinct kinds.

It is by understanding the lawlike generalizations and typical history and development that characterize members of the kind that one brings in under the extension members of the kind who are never a perfect fit with the arbitrary good specimen. A banana is a banana even if it has brown spots. The epistemic task of making the judgment that a given individual is a member of a particular natural kind is not a matter of pure deductive logic; it is not a matter of including individuals that have the necessary and sufficient predicates in the class and eliminating those that do not. It is accomplished in part by analogy, in part by deduction, and in part by the convergence of multiple modes of investigation—sensory, social, and scientific. Yet judging that an individual is a member of a kind is an utterly simple and basic epistemic task. I see a tree. I walk a hundred yards and I see another tree that looks just like it. Both are unique and have their differences, but I judge that they are the same kind of thing. I am able to discern that they are differentiated from the rest of reality as something, that is, each is an elm tree. Even children know how to make judgments of kind and identity. Grandma is still Grandma, even if she is sick and old.

Medicine, as a practice, is premised on the idea that losing one or another feature that is typical of the human natural kind does not render one a different kind of thing, but a damaged member of the kind in need of healing and restoration. One reaches out to help precisely because one recognizes both the humanness of the sick person and the fact that some characteristic feature is no longer functioning perfectly well. Denying the humanness of fetuses and the severely demented is not an attractive option for those who want to hold that only some members of the human natural kind have Dignity. It seems to entail the judgment that at least some sicknesses exclude one from the kind, and this undermines the moral foundation for the practice of medicine.

One final move would be to argue that there simply is no such thing as intrinsic value—that all values are attributed. The notion that nothing has value except from the perspective of a valuer suggests the famous view of Protagoras that "man is the measure of all things."[22] But certainly there can be no more anthropocentric view of the universe than this; no grosser form of speciesism than the view that no species has value except that conferred upon it by human evaluation. Obviously, human beings attribute value to many things. But the notion that a thing has intrinsic value does not preclude the possibility that human beings might attribute other values to it. Conversely, the fact that value might be attributed to a thing by a human valuer does not preclude the logical possibility that it might also have intrinsic value.

The view that nothing has intrinsic value is precisely the one that environmental ethicists are trying to counter. Yet other problems arise in ethics without a theory of intrinsic value. In human interaction, the possibility of ethics is radically threatened by such a position. If there is no reason why one must respect the interests of a person, then that person has no moral claims on anyone else, and no protection. Even an intersubjective attribution of intrinsic value to a person in an "as if" construction would not be a sustainable way out of this problem. If one were to build an ethic upon the premise that "we should all act as if there were an intrinsic value to being human and act accordingly even though, enlightened by philosophy, we know that there really is no intrinsic value to anything," one would still be left with the problem and having to give a reason to behave in such an "as if" fashion. This leads to the convoluted conundrum that deception and/or self-deception is the basis for morality, and would still leave one open to the arbitrary whims of whoever's preferences are eventually codified as the "as if" true moral precepts and would leave all persons constantly susceptible to arbitrary changes in these precepts.[23] Ultimately, if one is to be concerned about the interests of a person, this must be founded upon a respect for some sort of value inherent in the person whose interests they are. This is the value I have called intrinsic dignity.

NOTES

1. "Universal Declaration of Human Rights," available from www.un.org/Overview/rights.html.

2. "Convention for the Protection of Human Rights and Dignity of the Human Being with Regard to the Application of Biology and Medicine: Convention on

Human Rights and Biomedicine," Council of Europe Treaty no. 164, available from http://conventions.coe.int/Treaty/EN/CadreListeTraites.htm.

3. Ronald Dworkin, *Taking Rights Seriously* (Cambridge, MA: Harvard University Press, 1977), 198–99.

4. Daniel P. Sulmasy, "Death and Human Dignity," *Linacre Quarterly* 61 (November 1994): 27–36; Sulmasy, "Death with Dignity: What Does It Mean?" *Josephinum Journal of Theology* 4 (1997): 13–23; Sulmasy, "Healing the Dying: Spiritual Issues in the Care of the Dying," in *The Health Professional as Friend and Healer*, ed. J. Kissel and D. C. Thomasma (Washington, DC: Georgetown University Press, 2000), 188–97.

5. Daniel P. Sulmasy, "Death, Dignity, and the Theory of Value," *Ethical Perspectives* (2003): 103–18.

6. Noah M. Lemos, "Value," in *The Cambridge Dictionary of Philosophy*, ed. Robert Audi (New York: Cambridge University Press, 1995), 829–30.

7. Immanuel Kant, *Groundwork for the Metaphysics of Morals*, Ak 429, trans. James W. Ellington (Indianapolis, IN: Hackett, 1981), 36.

8. Holmes Rolston III, *Environmental Ethics* (Philadelphia: Temple University Press, 1988), 116.

9. Credit for initiation of the discussion of natural kinds is usually given to Saul Kripke, in his two essays, "Identity and Necessity," in *Identity and Individuation*, ed. Milton K. Munitz (New York: New York University Press, 1971), 135–64, and "Naming and Necessity," in *Semantics of Natural Language*, ed. Gilbert Harman and Donald Davidson (Dordrecht, Neth.: D. Reidel, 1972), 253–355. For a good contemporary approach to the concept of natural kinds, see David Wiggins, *Sameness and Substance* (Cambridge, MA: Harvard University Press, 1980), 77–101, and his *Sameness and Substance Renewed* (Cambridge: Cambridge University Press, 2001).

10. William Harper, "Natural Kind," in *The Cambridge Dictionary of Philosophy*, ed. Robert Audi (Cambridge: Cambridge University Press, 1995), 519–20. See also Wiggins, *Sameness and Substance*, and Baruch Brody, *Identity and Essence* (Princeton, NJ: Princeton University Press, 1980), 130–33.

11. Wiggins, *Sameness and Substance*, 169.

12. For a discussion of the concept of dispositional predicates in relation to natural kinds and ethical theory, see Anthony J. Lisska, *Aquinas's Moral Theory: An Analytic Reconstruction* (Oxford: Clarendon Press of Oxford University Press, 1996), 96–100.

13. Wiggins, *Sameness and Substance*, 132–33.

14. Ibid., 103–4.

15. Besides Kripke and Wiggins (see note 9) and Brody (see note 10), another very important figure in these arguments has been Hilary Putnam. See, for example, "Is Semantics Possible?" in *Mind, Language, and Reality: Philosophical Papers*, vol. 2 (Cambridge: Cambridge University Press, 1975), 50–63.

16. See Lisska, note 12, above.

17. Sulmasy, "Death and Human Dignity," "Death with Dignity," and "Healing the Dying."

18. Immanuel Kant, "The Metaphysics of Morals, Part II: The Metaphysical Principles of Virtue," Ak 462, in *Ethical Philosophy*, trans. James W. Ellington (Indianapolis, IN: Hackett, 1983), 127.

19. Boethius, *Contra Eutychen et Nestorium*, III, in *Boethius: The Theological Tractates*, trans. H. F. Stewart, E. K. Rand, and S. J. Tester (Cambridge, MA: Harvard University Press, 1973), 72–129. This work is also known as *De persona et duabus naturis*, ch. 1, *Patrologia Latina* 64, 1343, and is quoted in Thomas Aquinas, *Summa Theologiae* I., Blackfriars ed. (New York: McGraw-Hill, 1964), q. 29, a1.

20. Wiggins, *Sameness and Substance*, 174.

21. John Searle, *Intentionality: An Essay in the Philosophy of Mind* (New York: Cambridge University Press, 1983), 7.

22. This fragment comes from his book *On Truth*. The exact quote (in English translation) is, "Of all things the measure is man: of existing things, that they exist; of nonexistent things, that they do not exist." See *An Introduction to Early Greek Philosophy*, ed. John Manley Robinson (Boston: Houghton Mifflin, 1968), 245. The precise meaning is far from obvious, and I am using it here in one possible sense.

23. John A. Rist, *Real Ethics: Rethinking the Foundations of Morality* (Cambridge: Cambridge University Press, 2002), 20–24.

5

On Being True to Form

Margaret E. Mohrmann

> Autonomy is not the freedom to will one thing one moment and
> another the next. It is the freedom to establish an identity and
> maintain integrity.
>
> —Hessel Bouma et al.

This chapter focuses on the subject of integrity, considered from a Christian theological perspective and, ultimately, in relation to the concerns and methods of bioethics. Although not an arm of theological ethics, bioethics does bear some resemblance to a close cousin of theological ethics, ancient Greek philosophical ethics: bioethics, though neither eudaemonistic nor centered on individual character, tends toward the practical (multiple theories notwithstanding) and is formulated for a limited, even elite, portion of the population. That is, bioethics speaks to the doers of medicine, the practitioners and policymakers, but rarely, if at all, to the "done-to."

A serious consideration of integrity, however, pushes us to contemplate precisely the condition of those acted upon by medicine: patients, consumers, research subjects, and even, in these days, medical professionals. An exploration of integrity should help us explicate how persons who take their ills to medicine or who make medical decisions for themselves or their dependents, and who seek at the same time to be faithful—to themselves, to those they love, to God—may and do exhibit and maintain integrity.

To begin, I offer a twofold working definition of integrity, theologically understood:

(1) We say that a human being has or displays integrity insofar as she is consistently true—physically, mentally, spiritually—both to the intentional design of her divine creation and to the trajectory of her ongoing formation toward God.

(2) We also say that human beings have integrity in the sense that what we, for rhetorical convenience, refer to as the "parts" of a person—body, mind, soul, spirit—comprise, in actuality, one being, a single unity and not a hierarchically ordered conglomerate.

The first definition I shall call integrity as *consistency*, or a sort of sameness; the second, integrity as *oneness*, or unity. In order to deconstruct (and defend) each of these it is necessary to include an exploration of some aspects of the evolved usage of the word *integrity*.[1]

Integrity as Consistency

The immediate Latin source of the English word *integrity* is *integritas*, a noun that seems to have come into being in order to name the characteristic of a person or thing accurately described by the adjective *integer*. *Integer* itself is a second-order word, composed of the negating particle *in* attached to a form of the verb *tangere*, to touch. *Integer* fundamentally then means untouched, in the sense of being unaltered from some earlier or original state; its usage implies that the intactness of that original state is desirable and, in addition, that the original state is good, even perfect. This sense of being untouched is the basis for *integer*'s two categories of definition: one as spotless, unblemished, pure; the other as whole or entire, with nothing missing.

The ideas of purity and of the maintenance of an inherent intactness are strongly present in ancient Latin uses of *integer* and *integritas*, as can be seen in early, more concrete use of the words in reference to reproduced texts and their faithfulness to their originals. The definition quickly evolved to a more abstract application to persons and their reliable adherence to their original forms, thus giving the terms the strongly moral connotations that we now associate with our English word *integrity*. This sense of fidelity to an ideal form grounds not only the primary moral definition, in classical Latin, of *integritas* as moral uprightness but also the connotation of reliable constancy over time that distinguishes *integritas* from some other descriptors of moral goodness. The person of integrity is predictably true to form: even in the absence of a superficial uniformity of action, an underlying rationale—a consistent strand of commitment, adherence, and direction—imparts a reliability to that person's behavior and responses, often observable by others who can then recognize and name that quality of consistency or sameness as integrity.

The idea of "sameness," in this instance connoting equivalence more than constancy, is also the root meaning of the word *identity,* an observation that may enhance our comprehension of the meanings that integrity bears. *Identity* is derived, probably through the mediation of a French form of the word, from *identitas,* an interesting linguistic construction appearing in late Latin. English etymological dictionaries claim that *identitas* seems to have been invented—much as *integritas* was, but a good bit later and more selectively—in order to have a Latin noun that would denote sameness as equivalence. The declinable demonstrative pronoun *idem,* meaning "the same," had no qualitative counterpart. Dictionaries of classical Latin contain no word that conveys the sense of same*ness*, the quality of being the same; none of them lists the word *identitas.* The ancient Latin vocabulary does include the word *identidem,* an adverb thought to be an elided compound of *idem et idem* ("the same and the same"), translated as "repeatedly" or "again and again." *Identidem* led linguists to surmise that the *identi-* root is the combining form of *idem,* but there are no other *identi-* words in classical Latin.

Identitas appears to have been coined by Christian writers in late antiquity who were seeking a language with which to explain that the persons of the Trinity, even though we may speak of them in different ways, even with different names, are in truth the same.[2] The earliest recorded use of the word is in an anti-Arian tract written late in the fourth century by the Roman Christian rhetorician, Marius Victorinus (*Adv. Arium* 1.48, 1.59). By the Scholastic period, the definitions of *identitas* (or *idemptitas,* as it occasionally appears, showing more clearly its origin in *idem*), as collated in dictionaries of medieval ecclesiastical Latin, resembled closely current connotations of *identity*; its use to denote a quality of the Trinity had become only a technical subset of the primary definition: sameness of quality or attributes.[3]

Identity's characterization as sameness and integrity's as consistency beg a question for each word: "Same as what?" and "Consistent with what?" In very many ways, I am not the same person I was fifty years ago, or even twenty years ago, nor are my actions now entirely consistent with my actions then. Yet I have identity, and I claim integrity. What, then, is the standard in relation to which I profess sameness and consistency? The origins and evolved definitions of both identity and integrity push back to a basic construal of a human being as starting out with or, more accurately, being created as a particular thing, in a particular form that then serves as answer to the tacit questions. I have identity because, however much I have developed over time, I am still the same created person; I have integrity because the conduct of my life is consistent with the way I was created to live.

Most of the ancient classical thinkers who used the word *integritas* and certainly the early Christian thinkers who found *identitas* a helpful term believed that divine intentionality, of a more or less anthropomorphic sort, was at work in the creation of human beings, whether the creating act was understood as a dispersal of the Stoic *logos*, as an emanation from the Platonic *nous*, or as a deliberate work of God effected through the *logos,* who at a time in history had appeared in the created world as the human Jesus. The intentionality meant that human beings were created in this way and not that; creation imparted a specific form to humanness generally and to each human being in particular.

Implicit in this notion of an ideal created form—the intactness of which determines whether one is *integer* or not—is the idea, for Christian and non-Christian thinkers alike, that the divinely intended form of the person is altogether good. This is why, in common parlance, integrity, like its congener *integritas* in ancient usage, does not denote the reliable consistency of character of someone who habitually does evil. We may, and do, say disparagingly that a predictably annoying or overtly immoral person acts "true to form," but we would not seriously refer to such a person as having integrity in his or her actions. The phrase used as criticism is not the sense of being true to form that integrity bears and, in fact, suggests ironic censure precisely of the form that the person has adopted to substitute for the way he or she was designed to be. In contrast, the constancy that is called integrity, or the sameness that characterizes an integrated identity, is a mark of goodness because the referent for that consistency, that sameness, is the unblemished (*integer*) goodness of the person as created.

Creation is not the only way in which human beings are formed. Another, equally vital sense of formation has to do with the development of the nascent ideal form into that of a mature adult human being. A newborn has a profound sort of "integrity," an undeniable singleness of purpose, a smooth congruence of inner need and outer expression. Nevertheless, although we may honor and admire that instinctual integration of impulses, it would be frivolous to call it integrity in any fully human or moral sense. Clearly, then, there must be some notion of development, of ongoing formation—even, given our theological interests, reformation—that is important to the acquisition and expression of integrity, completely understood. For the sake of clarity in what is to come, I shall refer to the first sense of formation simply as *creation* and the second sense, the ongoing process, as *formation*, a usage that connects us to the sophisticated understandings of formation, particularly character formation, developed in both philosophical and religious schools of thought. Formation in this latter sense is as significant to an understanding of the human being, especially in relation to the concerns of medicine and bioethics, as is the claim that persons must refer to their ideal created form, and thus to originating divine intentions for human life, when considering the nature and maintenance of their integrity.

To begin, it is helpful to distinguish formation from education, even while acknowledging that the two processes may well be complementary, or even be two aspects of the same general system. The distinction is that education can be understood, rather Socratically, as a method of bringing out, of educing what is there in a person as potential. Formation, on the other hand, is a matter of giving form to that which is disordered or, perhaps better, not yet ordered.

In its narrower, more pedagogical sense, formation refers to the method by which a person is prepared for a particular task or is made capable of functioning in a particular role. One forms, as well as educates, priests, soldiers, nurses, and doctors in a process that moves beyond the knowledge content of those crafts to the moral content of the practices—the obligations entailed, the demands imposed—and thus to the moral formation of the practitioners. To form is not merely to cultivate or develop, but to mold, to prepare, to realize. Moreover, it is generally the case that one is formed toward something, some telos, some ideal shape or condition. It is through formation that one is helped to acquire certain dispositions or virtues and thus to become a particular kind of person progressing on the moral journey toward perfection of conduct and of humanness.[4]

However, formation, like education, cannot be understood only as the result of explicit external assistance or guidance. For one thing, formation is a further development of the originally given form and thus depends significantly on what has been given and not solely on the efforts of the guiding master or teacher.

For another—this is a point especially relevant to the topic of integrity—it seems to be the case that our formation into mature persons who are capable (or not) of displaying integrity is, for the most part, a consequence of our life experiences, situations, and relationships, at least as much as it is the result of a deliberate process of formation. Our original, created form of humanness enters on the process of further molding almost from the moment of our births. I am a pediatrician; what has pleased me most about the practice of pediatrics is the privileged position from which to observe the development of children from newborns to young adults, a development that is clearly not only physical growth, neurological maturation, and intellectual expansion but also moral formation. Like these other modes of development, moral formation can happen well or poorly. We are formed for good or for ill by what we see and hear and do, by the people we find ourselves with or choose to be with, by the situations—both mundane and critical—that come upon and engage us.

Aristotle knew this; he emphasized that attainment of a life of virtue required not only that the aspirant be "well brought up" but also that he be constantly in the company of other well-formed persons, so that even casual encounters would be positively formative. St. Paul knew this: "Whatever is true, whatever is honorable, whatever is just . . . if there is any excellence, if there is anything worthy of praise, think about these things" (Phil. 4.8). With each event or encounter, with each interaction or choice, another step is taken along some path of formation. Part of the purpose of education and the dominant purpose of deliberate processes of formation are to ensure that the inevitable formation be good, first, in that it is true both to the original divine good intention and to the desired and desirable goal of more nearly perfect goodness and, second, in that it is open to continuing divine guidance in order to ensure the good direction of the path.

Formation, theologically understood, is directed toward the realization of the ideal endowment given in creation. But it is also important to note that, however complete the original created design, ongoing formation is always necessarily not only individual but also contingent and partial. There are ways of saying this in religious language. One speaks of different people being at different places on their moral and spiritual "journeys," of there being many paths by which to come to and to know God, even of the various ways in which the human propensity to sin mars the original perfect form and impedes attempts to continue on the trajectory of divine formation. Despite many important and fundamental similarities among human beings—religious people tend to believe that God is, above all, consistent— we are neither created exactly the same nor formed exactly the same.

The implications of this model of creation and formation for a theological conception of integrity as a quality of human beings are many. Understanding integrity as "being true to form" includes the acknowledgment that we have been and are still being formed. Thus integrity is a constant term for a shifting ground, because formation is dynamic and continuous. Being true to one's original form as it has developed over time will not always look like someone else's fidelity, except in the broadest strokes, nor always look like internal consistency, at least not without further investigation.

A faithful expression of my integrity, were I, say, faced with a request to give one of my kidneys to a family member, might be quite different from that of someone else—with different experiences, resources, obligations, expectations, and so on—facing a similar request. Moreover, my demonstrations of integrity might vary considerably in different situations; my willingness to donate an organ might change at various points in my life as the nature of my obligations to particular others and to myself alters over time.

Being true to form does not imply a predetermined rigidity of response or action, in which one can play only the notes written on the page if one wishes to be part of the music. A better metaphor is dance: having and displaying integrity is more a matter of being able to move in ways that are consistent with the originating and developing themes of our lives. Teachers, guides, and practice make us better dancers because they help us listen more carefully and follow the music we hear more confidently. We learn which movements fit the rhythms and which do not. There is rarely just one way to enact an excellent dance to fit a particular melody—and sometimes, when we have learned to hear the music more clearly, to understand it more deeply, we find that we have to change our steps.[5]

Integrity understood as consistency has to be something other than the sort of foolish consistency against which Emerson warned us so cogently, something other than superficial sameness. The constancy of integrity is in respect to something fundamental and unchanging, not necessarily to the way I understood my situation yesterday or last year. The uniformity of integrity, as of identity, is not a lockstep obligation to make the same choices repeatedly, *identidem*; it is, rather, consistency as the ability to remain true to the same form and direction that define, determine, and identify our lives, while responding differentially according to the light of continuous learning and shaping, continually changing situations and perspectives. As the writer to the Hebrews tells us (13.8), "Jesus Christ is the same today and yesterday and forever," but the gospels show that Jesus was also differentially responsive to the situations in which he found himself.[6]

The consistency of integrity is not inflexibility; it is godliness. Understanding ourselves theologically to be called to become more and more like God, we recognize the imperfection, the partiality of what we can grasp at any point along our way from original design to completion in God. Our godliness does not imply that we have reached the perfection to which we aspire, only that we are on the right path, guided by the illumination available in each moment to discern the lineaments of the route, to keep us true to form, faithful to the origin, direction, and goal of the journey. Complicating the claim of Bouma et al. in this chapter's epigraph, that "autonomy is not the freedom to will one thing one moment and another the next," is the recognition that my ongoing formation toward God may mean that, at times, I shall be obliged to will one thing one moment and another the next. This, too, can be integrity.

The argument is not that God is changing with each moment, that God acts or guides erratically, but rather that my understanding of what it is to be godly, to follow God's shaping guidance, changes as I understand more about the situation, more about myself in it, more about God's call to me. Thus, a theological anthropology may call on the ethics of medicine not only to honor a person's right to make decisions for herself, even if that entails an unaccountable change of mind, but also to recognize and support the possibility of true integrity in such a move.

This understanding of integrity's "sameness" serves as yet another argument against some clinicians' tendency to presume, given enough experience with a patient, that they know how that person will respond to a particular diagnosis or what that person's decision will be about a recommended course of treatment—a presumption that can lead to the presentation of an unnecessarily limited array of options, to half-truths and unbridgeable communication gaps, among other things. Moreover, this construal speaks against the assumptions we make about ourselves and the nature of the consistency to which we aspire. I have not yet experienced serious illness in myself (see chapter 6, by Suzanne Holland). I can and do make assumptions about what I shall want or choose when I am, eventually, faced with decisions about chemotherapy or dialysis, heart surgery or life support. But I do not really know how God will form me—what I shall learn, what new wisdom I shall acquire, how I shall change—between now and then, or in and through the experience itself. I believe that the formation to come will be in harmony with what has gone before, but I cannot know now what I do not know now. Therefore I must be open to what my ongoing development will teach me, open to learning something perhaps oddly new and unforeseen. The nonstatic nature of the formation with which integrity must be consistent, and therefore of integrity itself, indicates that there may be quite good reasons to change one's mind, from time to time, precisely in order to maintain integrity—and identity.

Integrity as Oneness

Consistency is not the only characteristic of the moral content of integrity that needs to be considered in relation to bioethics. Further investigation of *integer* and *integritas* in Latin Christian writing and of some of the earliest uses of "integrity" in English leads us to another connotation of integrity that is of particular relevance to our discussions. Integrity, in Christian usage, implies not only constancy but also oneness, as becomes clear from a brief historical survey of Christian literature.

The earliest Christian uses of *integritas* centered almost entirely on a definition that was not the predominant usage in non-Christian Latin, that of chastity, the integrity of the untouched female body. Although chastity was certainly attributed to and praised in males, the word used in the male context was always one of the several other Latin words that mean chastity. *Integritas* was used to refer solely to women's chastity, apparently because of the entrenched physicalist assumption that women forfeit their integrity—are no longer spotless, no longer whole—when they are penetrated during the act of intercourse, whereas men do not give up their integrity by engaging in sex as the penetrators, even if they lose their virginity or abandon chastity thereby.

It is not until the late fourth century, first with Ambrose and then, more elaborately, in the writings of Augustine, that we can discern in Christian usage a moral sense of *integritas* that goes beyond female chastity, recaptures the broader classical understanding, and looks toward the later Christian and eventual English connotations of consistent moral uprightness and probity. Both Ambrose and Augustine make the specific point that, when the chips are down and choices must be made, *integritas* of the mind or the soul must be preferred to *integritas* of the body. Specifically, their point is that, if the choice is between forswearing allegiance to God and being raped, it is better to endure the rape. It is even preferable, according to Augustine, to allow the rape than to tell a lie in order to avoid it.

It is worth looking at Augustine's point in more detail, because it takes us toward an important understanding of integrity as oneness, a sense of the word that underlies both its development within Christian thought and its current usage in English. In his essay "On Lying," Augustine writes:

> there is no purity [*pudicitia*] of the body except as it depends on the *integritas* of the mind; this *integritas* being broken, the other must needs fall, even though it seem intact. . . . By no means, therefore, must

the mind corrupt itself by a lie for the sake of the body, which it knows remains incorrupt if incorruptness does not depart from the mind. . . . Thus, since no one doubts that the mind is better than the body, to *integritas* of body we ought to prefer *integritas* of mind, which can be preserved forever. But who would say that the mind of one who tells a lie has its integrity [*integrum esse*]? (*De mendacio* 1.10)

Notable here is Augustine's working through an understanding of the interconnectedness of body and mind, using a relatively new idea within Christianity[7] that somehow the body's integrity, understood as its state of being pure and inviolate, is not an isolated phenomenon but is intimately related to—dependent upon, Augustine would say—the integrity of the *anima*, the mind or the soul. What allows Augustine to make this move is a connotation, not fully elaborated in the old Latin definitions but gradually brought out by Christian thinkers, of *integer* and *integritas* as oneness, singleness. The sense of the adjective *integer* as whole or entire supports a concept of unity; to be *integer*, to have *integritas*, is to be a whole not in the sense of a collection of multiple parts but in the sense of being one thing.

This connotation of oneness is corroborated by the word choices made by some of the earliest English users of "integrity." In the authorized, or King James Version (KJV), of the bible, compiled only 150 years after the first known appearance of "integrity" in English, the translators' use of the word indicates their understanding of its meanings. Comparing instances of "integrity" in the KJV with the corresponding Latin passages of Jerome's Vulgate, one finds that, in each instance, "integrity" translates a word or idea that Jerome rendered as *innocentia* or *simplicitas*. Outside the books of Job and Psalms, where Jerome uses these two words interchangeably, the only Latin word corresponding to "integrity" is *simplicitas*. Whereas *innocentia* connotes blamelessness, *simplicitas*' primary definition is singleness of nature, unity. The early seventeenth-century translators' decision to express primarily this concept as "integrity"—for example, in no instance in the KJV does "integrity" refer to female chastity—signifies the weight given to oneness, singleness of nature as a defining characteristic of integrity as it entered English usage.

One implication of this understanding is that theologically, and despite all pressures to the contrary, integrity resists a virtually dualist definition that would read the oneness of the human person as a matter of two (or more) parts being held together well, that is, in the correct order. Augustine takes us in this dualist direction—not surprisingly, perhaps, given his

Platonic predilections—when, in the lines from *De mendacio* cited earlier, he speaks of the mind's superiority to the body, in phrases that imply that corruption of the mind will destroy the body, but loss of merely physical integrity need not impair the soundness of a good mind. Echoes of that sort of insidious dualism, in latter days given shelter by Cartesian formulations, can be found in such familiar religious phrases as the one that defines chastity as having the body in the soul's keeping, without attention to the reciprocal idea that the soul and the mind are also and significantly in the body's keeping.

Although I would not deny the heuristic value of that kind of trope—the body in the soul's keeping—I would press the point that a theological anthropology, especially one speaking to bioethics, cannot afford a lapse into the dualism lurking in such a statement, which may too casually allow things to be done to the body on the premise that the mind or the soul, and therefore the person, need not be harmed thereby. The oneness of integrity demands that we take the possible effect on the whole person of bodily alteration or violation as seriously as Augustine, and we, take the ability of the mind to "rise above" what is happening to the body.

Augustine's discussion of the primacy of the mind's integrity represented a salutary change from the prevailing view that, no matter the woman's role, rape invariably and permanently destroyed her integrity—and therefore she may as well die—but it nevertheless runs the significant risk of suggesting that nothing of consequence has happened when it appears that the body alone has been violated. Moreover, Augustine, in insisting on the primacy of mind—an emphasis so characteristic of his time—does not help us contemplate situations in which disruptions of mental or spiritual integrity may be called for in order to preserve physical integrity, or to consider that allowing such psychic violations could be morally obligatory in certain circumstances. I am thinking of a situation, for example, in which telling a lie could be necessary to save one's own life, a life whose continued existence may be required for the preservation of other lives. It would seem that an understanding of the complexities that comprise our formation as people of integrity could construe lying in such a situation as an affirmation of integrity in the most complete sense.

The oneness of integrity forces us to take entirely seriously things that are done to bodies as well as things that violate minds, precisely because each sort of action is done to persons, who are not body *plus* mind and soul and spirit, but are body/mind/soul/spirit: all one, nonhierarchically integrated, *integer*. Christians have managed, with more or less success, to comprehend

Trinitarian thinking about God; holding on to monotheism while believing that God is three should be good preparation, and a helpful analogy, for insisting on the oneness of the human being that integrity denotes.

Speaking to Bioethics

Much of the theory and practice of bioethics has long been directed, and understandably so, toward critical issues in medical care: those arising at the extremes of life or from encounters with patients who can no longer make decisions or never could, or the like. But this focus has left bioethics with a few sizeable and troublesome blind spots:

(1) Having convinced medical professionals to allow patients to be the decision makers, in the name of autonomy or respect for persons, bioethics nevertheless provides little or no guidance for patients making decisions. The ethical theories and moral deliberations of bioethics are generally about dilemmas plaguing medical professionals and policymakers, not about quandaries faced by patients and their families. Attention to patients as persons seeking to maintain their integrity by being consistent, being "true to form," suggests that bioethics should consider, and find helpful ways to speak to, the moral obligations—and conflicts among moral obligations—borne by autonomous medical decision makers.

(2) Despite the fact that outpatient generalist practice constitutes, by far, the majority of medical encounters, bioethics spares relatively little time or thought for the issues of primary care medicine: the mundane complaints and quotidian concerns, the efforts to preserve health and prevent or delay decline, the day-to-day working together of patients and doctors outside of hospitals. Concern for integrity has implications not only for critical medical decisions but also—and perhaps more crucially given their frequency and potential effects on the ongoing formation of body, mind, and spirit—for choices relating to diet, physical activity, smoking, stress levels, family relationships, childbearing and rearing, use of alcohol and other drugs, and so on. These matters occupy a significant part, even the majority of a generalist's time and attention. Medical education covers most of them repeatedly and at length. But bioethics, for the most part, does not contribute to the discussion. An

understanding of integrity as oneness suggests that health should be of as much interest to the ethics of medicine as is disease and disability. Physicians and patients would benefit from bioethics' attention to the ordinary decisions of living that enact our stewardship of ourselves as embodied.

(3) Although I can only gesture toward the topic here, it is important to raise the subject, also generally neglected by bioethics, of the integrity—physical, mental, spiritual, unitary—of health care practitioners. Just as bioethics tends to focus on critical issues in medicine, it also tends to focus on medicine's moral obligations to its patients. With the advent of interest in organizational ethics, plus a significant increase in nursing scholarship about such issues as the prevalence of moral distress among health care providers, there is ample opportunity for bioethics to attend to the moral well-being as well as the moral formation of clinicians. The issues vary from the problems of maintaining professional and personal integrity in the face of the commodification of medical practice or the institutional routinization of nursing practice to that of recognizing violations of practitioners' physical integrity—and, consequently, mental and spiritual integrity—that may be perpetrated by some forms of training and some demands of practice.[8] A theological anthropology for bioethics can call the discipline to recognize and honor, to speak to and reason about, the integrity of *all* persons engaged in clinical encounters, in medical and nursing education, in medical and nursing research.

This final claim, while certainly justified, raises an additional question about these and other neglected but troublesome issues in medicine, specifically in relation to the role of theological inquiry: Are such matters entirely within the purview of bioethics, as the field is currently conceived, or might they be better construed as issues about which theologians and theological ethicists should be prepared to puzzle, confer, and exhort? That is, perhaps the project of constructing a theological anthropology for bioethics should be taken to be not so much a contribution to bioethics, calling it to expand its borders and deepen its perspective, but as an initial effort at elaborating—in full communication with but parallel to bioethics—a theological ethics of medicine, health, illness, disability, and dying for the benefit of believers who may be or become medicine's patients, practitioners, administrators, and policymakers.

NOTES

I am grateful to the Georgetown University Center for Clinical Bioethics, especially its director, Carol R. Taylor, CSFN, for the opportunity to participate in the project that resulted in this book, and to the conferees, whose lively and insightful discussions have expanded my own horizons of thought.

1. In a recent paper I discuss the Latin origins and something of the history of Western Christian usage of the word *integrity*. I shall rehearse just enough of that in this paper to ground my arguments. For more detail, see Margaret E. Mohrmann, "Integrity: *Integritas, Innocentia, Simplicitas,*" *Journal of the Society of Christian Ethics* 24, 2 (2004): 25–37.

2. This process of back formation of new nouns from pronouns to serve the needs of Christian theology can also be seen in the coining in scholastic Latin of *quidditas*, "whatness," as well as the less common *haecceitas*, "thisness," neither of which is known to classical Latin.

3. See, for example, Albert Blaise, ed., *Dictionnaire Latin-Français des Auteurs Chretiens* (Turnhout, Belg.: Éditions Brepols, 1954), and D. R. Howlett, ed., *Dictionary of Medieval Latin from British Sources* (Oxford: Oxford University Press, 1997).

4. See the illuminating discussion of formation in the *Dictionnaire de Spiritualité* (Paris: Beauchesne, 1964), 5:696–99.

5. This metaphorical explanation of the flexibility of integrity bears a close resemblance to *finesse*, as it is discussed elsewhere in this volume by William Desmond, in chapter 3, who writes that "Finesse refers us to the concrete suppleness of living intelligence that is open, attentive, mindful, and attuned to the occasion in all its elusiveness and subtlety."

6. See Dietrich Bonhoeffer's explication of the ethical actions of Jesus as personal and situational in *Ethics* (New York: Macmillan, 1965), 84–85.

7. The idea can also be found in Ambrose's writing from roughly the same time: "That which is worthy is done not solely by the virginity of the flesh but also by the *integritas* of the mind." *De virginitate* 4.15. See also his praise of a maiden who chose to sacrifice her virginity rather than abandon her religious beliefs. *De virginibus* 2.4.

8. See, for example, Daniel F. Chambliss, *Beyond Caring: Hospitals, Nurses, and the Social Organization of Ethics* (Chicago: University of Chicago Press, 1996); Ann B. Hamric, "Moral Distress in Everyday Ethics," *Nursing Outlook* 48, no. 5 (2000): 199–201; and Margaret E. Mohrmann, "Professing Medicine Faithfully: Theological Resources for Trying Times," *Theology Today* 59, no. 3 (2002): 355–64.

CHAPTER

6

The Integrity Conundrum

Suzanne Holland

In bioethics the conversation on integrity most commonly takes place in research ethics. We are all loath to repeat the horrors of Tuskegee, and so we design research studies with what we hope is integrity—that is to say, we aim first of all to protect the dignity and vulnerability of the persons in our studies. This we do through informed consent and through the principle of autonomy. But little of this, while laudable, is helpful in the many cases that come to us outside of the research arena. By focusing on a particular case, I aim to excavate what integrity means in its theological context, as a way of thinking through issues in bioethics that seem to be connected by an invisible thread from our heads to our hearts.

I begin by exploring the roots of integrity itself. What are its origins? What kind of theological sense does it include? In other words, does integrity tell us anything critical about what it means to be a human being trying to sort out the conundrums life throws at us? Indeed, does it tell us anything at all about being a human person before God, and if it does, is this clarifying, or does it obfuscate even further? Is it a helpful concept as we sort through the practical muddles of bioethics? After examining the origins and context of integrity I consider the case of elective cosmetic surgery, specifically breast augmentation. I offer a framework for corporeal integrity that I hope goes some way toward helping sort out the ethics of elective surgical makeovers. In doing so, I attempt to integrate a theological ethics into a realm that has largely been the province of philosophical bioethics.[1]

Integrity in Historical and Etymological Context

The Oxford English Dictionary (OED) notes that integrity derives from the Latin adverb *integritas*, meaning "wholeness, entireness, completeness, chastity, purity, f. *integer, integr-* whole, INTEGER." Its earliest recorded usage seems to have been around 1420, and its evolution moved from a sense of material wholeness—the condition of having nothing taken away—to something undivided (1620), to "the condition of not being marred or violated . . . original perfect state" (1561, 1650), and then to the *moral sense* of the word, "unimpaired moral state; freedom from moral corruption; innocence, sinlessness," which the OED lists as obsolete. The moral sense appears in Calvin's *Institutes* (1561), for example, I.54: "In this integritie, man had freewil, whereby if he would he might haue attened eternall life." Undoubtedly, Calvin would have been influenced by Aquinas, and perhaps Augustine on this point.

The OED gives the common usage of integrity as "soundness of moral principle; the character of uncorrupted virtue, esp. in relation to truth and fair dealing; uprightness, honesty, sincerity." In the eighteenth and nineteenth centuries its usage is applied to "integrity of heart" (1795, Gentl. Mag. 543/1), and the notion that one tends to "trust in a person known to be of thorough integrity, that he will always be upright" (McCosh 1874). Although it lists the usage of innocence and sinlessness as being obsolete, the OED's inclusion of "the character of uncorrupted virtue" in common usage does appear rather closely related to the former, obsolete sense of integrity.

Whether the ancients thought of integrity as a virtue in itself, it is difficult to tell. Plato wrote about integrity in *The Republic* as the quality of the philosopher; however, when Aristotle wrote *Nichomachean Ethics,* he did not discuss integrity as among the virtues, unless it may have been one of the virtues for which he could not find a name, such as in his discussion of truthfulness, "the mean—also nameless—of which boastfulness is an extreme" (1127a/14). Aristotle's discussion of moral strength and moral weakness in Book VII in some ways resembles what we think of as integrity, and yet not. Integrity was probably a second-order virtue for Aristotle. Augustine, too, can be read as alluding to integrity when he reveals his struggles with his own concupiscence in his *Confessions*. Saint Thomas Aquinas equated virginity with moral integrity (*Summa Theologiae* 2-2, 152, 1-2). Thus we have the origins of the debate over flesh and reason that has troubled dogmatic theology from Augustine to Rahner.

In a theological sense, it is God who is the author of integrity. Perhaps integrity is another of the names for God, the whole One, the complete One—the One. If God is the only whole number, the original integer so to speak, it is easy to see how medieval theology made sense of integrity by positing that humankind had fallen away from our chance at original wholeness through the sin of Adam. Thus integrity had to be a state of purity and sinlessness, a state at which to aim, but one that would never be attained in this life. If, on the other hand, we see God not as the only whole, but as the author of every integer—every whole number (and integers are infinite)—then integrity opens up into a new dimension of possibility, as I discuss later.

On reflection, however, one might say that Aristotle was right in not naming integrity as a virtue, for what seems to distinguish it is not some characteristic we might then call virtuous, but the fact of indivisible coherence, the fact that one could have a kind of harmony of commitments and beliefs, that one would always choose to act in accord with this harmonious sense of self. Aristotle's sense of virtue as the mean between two extremes is "harmonious," we might say, with a view of integrity as that which gives us the capacity for this middle ground. As I have said, integrity as harmony and coherence is not inherently a virtue; it may lead one to choose a virtuous path—or put differently—it may equip one to choose the virtues, though such a conclusion does not have to follow from the premise.

In a formalistic sense, a person of integrity may choose vices as well as virtues, for integrity cannot guarantee the content of our commitments. In this view, we would have to allow that someone such as Osama bin Laden, for example, might have a great deal of integrity. Assuming that bin Laden is not psychotic (for then he would have no unity of personality, or integrity, from a psychological perspective), then who is to say that the choices this man makes to wage terrorist war on the West is any less a sign of integrity than the choices President Bush makes to wage war on Iraq? Or to use a more stark contrast, who is to say that bin Laden lacks integrity, while maintaining (as we certainly would) that Gandhi had it in spades? Why would we think of Dorothy Day or Mother Theresa as having had integrity, but not parents who give graduation gifts of breast enlargements to their teenage daughters? This is a clue that integrity must trigger for us something other than mere coherence, but how, and why?

Three Kinds of Alterations

I HAVE A CONFESSION TO MAKE: I have become addicted to reality television makeover shows. It began innocently enough with *Queer Eye for the Straight Guy*, mostly because I thought the premise was amusing: gay men spiffing up style-impaired heterosexuals. Then I began to watch nearly every episode of ABC's cosmetic surgery makeover show, *Extreme Makeover*. I found it had a numinous quality: It both attracted and repulsed me, and I knew I had become a makeover TV junkie. When my partner begged me to stop, I justified all of my reality television watching under vociferous and defensive protests: "It's research!" When Fox came out with its competing reality makeover show, *The Swan,* in which women are surgically altered and then compete against one another for a title and prizes (the ugly duckling loses), I thought we had reached an all-time cultural low. But still I watched. Perhaps I continue to watch because I too have been made over, though not in the way of *The Swan* and *Extreme Makeover*.

I spent much of 2003 in the office of a cosmetic/plastic surgeon; I had two elective surgeries to make my breasts look better and have become quite familiar with the panoply of alterations offered by cosmetic surgeons. It reminds me a little of going to the dressmaker with my mother, going in with a bolt of fabric and coming out with a beautiful dress. In truth, I secretly wish I had the money for liposuction, known in the vernacular as the "fat suck" operation. I would love for my legs to look twenty-something instead of forty-something. As it is, I am sure I never would have opened the door of a plastic surgeon's office had I not had breast cancer and lost both breasts to it. My reconstructed breasts do look better, but that's a relative assessment: they look better than my mastectomy scars, that is all.

BACK WHEN I WAS TWENTY-SOMETHING I volunteered at the spouse abuse center in my hometown. My job was to go the emergency room of the county hospital when women were admitted for battery, counsel them as to their options for safety, take pictures, and make sure a report got filed. It was never pretty. Once I met a woman, Cary, whose boyfriend had poured kerosene on her and set her on fire; she was black, but in the emergency room that night, she looked white. All of her skin had been peeled off from the flames. I never saw her again, but I knew that if she lived through that night she would likely have a future of painful reconstructive surgery. That was more than twenty years ago, yet I am sure that women like Cary appear today in every hospital emergency room in the country on any night of the week.

Not long ago I read that the National Coalition Against Domestic Violence (NCADV) has a direct services project called the Cosmetic and Reconstructive Support Program (CRS), which gives domestic abuse survivors free cosmetic and dental surgery so that they can make a fresh start. Survivors are matched to programs put together by cosmetic surgeons, dermatologists, and dentists to treat such women on a pro bono basis. In most cases, this means repair and reconstruction of broken, burned, or disfigured faces and dental work for broken teeth. In all cases, it means renewed self-esteem. I wish such a program had existed when Cary came into the hospital that night.

I HAVE A SIXTEEN-YEAR-OLD FRIEND I'll call Caitlin. Her mother, whom I will call Sandy, is a lifelong friend of mine. Sandy had breast augmentation surgery a few years ago. Among friends and family, Sandy's decision was privately tut-tutted: it was seen as hedonistic, self-indulgent, and self-centered; in short it met with resounding disapproval. (Among the same set of people, my decision to reconstruct my breasts was accepted, even admired.) Many times I have wondered how Sandy's decision to have surgically enlarged breasts has affected her daughter's sense of self as Caitlin finds her way through those painful teenage years of early sexuality.

Sandy and Caitlin do not live in California, but if they did, I wonder if Sandy and her husband would find themselves giving their daughter Southern California's most popular high school graduation gift of breast implants. "In California," writes Newhouse News Service reporter Kathleen O'Brien, "breast implants are reportedly the trendy high school graduation gift from parents."[2] Evidently, liposuction is not far behind. An often-cited statistic is that teenage cosmetic surgery nearly doubled from fewer than 14,000 to 24,623, between 1996 and 1998, according to data from the American Society of Plastic and Reconstructive Surgeons. The trend is growing, aided by the cultural message that "kids can, with enough money, change their bodies for the better."[3]

If it is true that kids are being encouraged—whether by cultural messages or by their parents—to "change their bodies for the better," buying breast augmentations and preventative Botox injections, while abused women apply for free cosmetic surgery to erase the damage done to their bodies by abusive spouses, and while "ordinary" women compete against one another on television to see whose surgical makeover renders them the most beautiful and who gets voted ugly duckling, well, I have to say that I find this all rather morally unsettling. What is it that unsettles me, I wonder? To answer this question I find myself turning to—as happens every semester of my teaching life—H. Richard Niebuhr's moral philosophy.

What Is Going On?

Since I have made hundreds of undergraduates answer moral dilemmas using Niebuhr's ethics of the fitting, it seems only "fitting" that I try it myself. Niebuhr counsels that in order to answer the central question of ethics, "What must I do?" one must first pose the question "what is going on?" The three scenarios I just described give content to this all-important question. What all three have in common is that we live in a time and place in which medicine has made it possible to alter the body with state-of-the-art technology. It is now safer than ever before to get cosmetic surgical alterations. Not only is it safer, medicine has been harnessed to the market so that cosmetic surgery is widely available, and if it is not widely affordable, it can be obtained the American way—through credit financing. In short, this is "what is going on."

Niebuhr's second-order question, "what is the fitting response?" is much harder to answer, but I suspect that it entails coming to grips with integrity, if not moral integrity, then at least, in terms of cosmetic alterations, corporeal integrity. Concretely, did Sandy's decision to augment her breasts have corporeal integrity? Did mine? Was either decision a fitting response? In order to answer this we need to explore what Niebuhr meant by the fitting response.

This concept of Niehuhr's necessitates the realization that everything we do is subject to being qualified by the communities of which we are a part and by the causes to which we are loyal. In fact, that is how he defines what it means to be a Christian—one who is loyal to the causes of Jesus Christ.

Now, we may be loyal to many causes, even to conflicting causes. One may find oneself, for example, an evangelical Christian, and a gay or lesbian person in a committed sexual relationship. The point is that while we often have many loyalties—church, school, family, job, Little League, hospice volunteer work—there is one loyalty beyond all these that completes us. For the theist, that loyalty is to God, "the One beyond the many," as Niebuhr so beautifully put it.[4] It is this One who drives us beyond the chaos and cacophony of our diverse and particular loyalties and toward universal community.

Niebuhr allows that we do, of course, make choices that are limited to one or another of our loyalties, or to one or another of our communities. In fact, we often make what we think are sincere and ethical choices, choices that speak of integrity. For example, the choice made by President Bush to go to war against Iraq may have been such a choice, and it is one that many Americans still find honorable, and even ethical. But in Niebuhr's terms we would have to say that it was a choice characterized by survivalist or "defense ethics," and thus could not be an *ethical* choice.

In other words, on a basic, almost existential level, we are confronted with two overarching worldviews, one of life and one of death—what Niebuhr referred to as the "mythology of death." If we choose, through the circumstances of our lives, to view the world suspiciously, as full of enemies, then we will also view God with suspicion, and our attitude may be one of hostility, or even unbelief. Then I will seek to protect my group or community or family from the enemies that I perceive are threatening it. If I fear annihilation, my "ethics" can only be one of defense or survival. As Niebuhr wrote, "Deep in our minds is the myth. . . . It appears as the story of the infinite progress of a particular species, this human kind, moving outward into space with its conquests, forward in time with victories over nature, but leaving behind in its past forgotten, dead generations. . . . It has scores of forms, no doubt, this mythology of death. But all its forms lead to the same interpretations in the present. . . . And all the forms lead to the ethos of defense, to the ethics of survival."[5] When I see death as the ultimate reality, my response to every situation will be qualified by that ultimate reality.

In Niebuhr's theocentric view, a response made out of fear of annihilation, while understandable, cannot be ethical, and here integrity comes into play. If I allow my responses to be qualified by an ethos of death, they will always be partial and not whole, for I have not then allowed my responses to be qualified by the Whole, the universal, and the infinite. In addition, as a responsible self in the world (and here Niebuhr meant, literally, the self-who-responds) I am very much a contingent self; I am in fact dependent upon others, upon the human community.

The fact of our existence as selves is this: there is no way to know myself as a subject except in relation to other selves. And for the theist, the self's very existence is radically contingent upon God the creator because it is God who gives coherence to the fragmented self. Niebuhr asks, "But what ties all these responsivities and responsibilities together, and where is the responsible *self* among all these roles played by the individual being?" And he answers, "To respond to the ultimate action in all responses to finite actions means to seek one integrity of self amidst all the integrities of scientific, political, economic, educational, and other cultural activities; it means to be one responding self amidst all the responses of the roles being played, because there is present to the self the One other beyond all the finite systems of nature and society."[6]

Niebuhr's articulation of self-in-relation to others, but more importantly in relation to God, is a bridge to the coherence of the inner and the outer. It reminds us that our actions are qualified by "the one universal society which has its center neither in me nor in any finite cause but in the Transcendent One."[7] So what is the fitting response with regard to the question of breast implantation? Was Sandy's response "fitting"? Was mine?

One way of arriving at an answer is to consider the source of the burdens each of us had to bear.[8] Obviously, I cannot really know the source of burden that Sandy carried, so I am aware that what I say here is merely speculative. In my eyes, Sandy always looked perfectly proportional to her five feet three inches and 110-pound frame, although she told me that she had felt dissatisfaction with her breast size for a number of years. So when she had enough money, Sandy got elective surgery that increased her breasts to a size C from a size A-plus. Sandy is thrilled with the results and purchased a new wardrobe that shows her new asset to best effect. She had felt burdened by having what she considered to be abnormally small breasts in a culture that doesn't value small breasts. Now Sandy feels that she "fits in" wherever she goes, especially with men. It seems clear that the original and ongoing source of Sandy's burden is external: prevailing social and cultural norms about female beauty. In Niebuhr's language we might say that Sandy operated under the mythology of death: she feared annihilation. That is to say, she feared invisibility, that she would not be seen or perhaps valued without conforming to the cultural norm.

What about me? In a real sense, I faced an issue of death from cancer, but the mythology of death had never been my ethos. Though I also had small breasts—approximately the same size as Sandy's—I did not feel the societal standard of beauty as one that caused me suffering. To be perfectly honest, I never felt particularly comfortable having small breasts, but I never seriously considered cosmetic enhancement surgery, and I had no desire to live in any body other than my own despite its imperfections. That is not to say that I don't work on my body; I go to the gym, I run, I try and watch my fat intake, and so on. But then, at age forty-six, I received a diagnosis of breast cancer. In order to maximize my chances of long-term survival, I had both breasts removed. Since the bilateral mastectomies removed both the current and future threat of cancer to a high percentage, I was able to elect reconstructive surgery at the same time as the mastectomies. When I ask myself what was the source of the burden I was made to bear, it seems crystal clear: cancer. With clothes on, my reconstructed breasts allow me to pass as "normal."

The fact that both of us want to pass as "normal" indicates to me the pervasiveness of the cultural standards of beauty in our society. Nonetheless, it does seem to be the case that the source of our decisions, Sandy's and mine, came from two different places. While I chose to restore my breasts to a very rough approximation of what I had before cancer claimed them, I did it as restoration of the original form rather than augmentation of it. It seems to me that Sandy had internalized the external cultural standards under which women in particular labor in this society; perhaps she simply chose not to fight against it anymore. One need only thumb through any popular magazine or turn on the television to see that women appear to be rewarded for having thin legs, large breasts, long silky (blonde) hair, and an ever-youthful appearance.

I do not fault Sandy's decision; it saddens me. It saddens me as I imagine what it conveys to Caitlin that her mother purchased large breasts and lives a happier life for it. And it saddens me when I juxtapose this reality against that of women who are disfigured from abuse, and whose faces will never be restored. I wonder how we can have lost our way so thoroughly. Margaret Mohrmann's discussion of integrity as "being true to form" (chapter 5) might be a helpful guide here, and it provides a nice bridge to Niebuhr's ethics of the fitting.

The Fitting Response: Being True to Form

In her chapter in this book, Mohrmann reminds us that the ancients, believing in the ideal created form, affirmed that one's original form was divinely created and wholly good. In this view, integrity is understood as consistency, as "being true to form." While attractive, one has to ask what virtue there is in slavish devotion to static and ideal form. Mohrmann answers that: "Integrity understood as consistency has to be something other . . . than superficial sameness. . . . The uniformity of integrity . . . is, rather, consistency as the ability to remain true to the same form and direction that define, determine, and identify our lives, while responding differentially according to the light of continuous learning and shaping, continually changing situations and perspectives."[9] In my case I think it is true that I had already come to terms with the corporeal form that was mine and had no plan to use surgery to alter it. When illness took part of my body, I used medical technology to restore the original form, which I had already affirmed as good. In Sandy's case, she used medical technology to try and alter her trajectory away from the divinely given form as good in itself. At some point, she had come to accept an ethos of threat and fear of annihilation, and her response was coherent with such an ethos. In this sense, it was a fitting response, but not a fully ethical response in the way that Niebuhr meant. To combine Mohrmann and Niebuhr, one might suggest that the real fitting response is "being true to form."

Virginia Ramey Mollenkott once wrote something to the effect that we know God in our bodies or we know God not at all.[10] This is a profound insight, and one that underpins my view of integrity. Integrity itself cannot be bifurcated—one sense of it for the body, and another for spirituality. For Christians, the Incarnation *is* the integration of body and spirit. The body is the intimate place of the divine, and it is where we integrate knowledge, perspective, emotion, virtues, and commitments. In other words, integrity is the wholeness that gives coherence to our lives as persons—and in my case, as a woman who believes in the One beyond the many.

Though most of us know right away when we are in the presence of someone who has integrity, what makes us so certain? The short answer, I think, is that the person appears to us to have a unity of character so that when she has a decision to make, we are sure that she will always act with as much honesty and as much truth as she is able to summon. We might say that she acts, as Mohrmann says, true to form, so that there is "a smooth congruence of inner need and outer expression."[11] The person of integrity acts this way consistently because she has done some kind of prior interior work and because she has cultivated the importance of listening for truth, listening for perspective. Thus she will move forward in her trajectory toward the One beyond the many with a coherence that affirms the goodness of her creation.

Part of the root of integer is *tangere*, Latin for "to touch," and thus integrity literally means: in + tangere = not to touch. The paradox is that, in order for one to have this unified completeness that we think of as integrity, it entails being utterly and completely "in touch."[12] In order to act from singleness of heart one needs to be in touch with the deepest parts of oneself; one must know the ways of the heart, which as scripture tells us, is "more devious than any thing." And one needs to be in touch with the wider world of which one is a part so that the self is not subject to the tyranny of the present moment, as Niebuhr might have said. He understood that human beings are fragmented: we have many loyalties and short attention spans. That is why Niebuhr insisted that only God unifies our many selves, by drawing us into God's cause—that which is universal, which is good for all humanity.

Feminists used to say that the personal is political, and that maxim seems apt to me in a discussion of enhancement technologies. Even though the issues of integrity I have been discussing appear to involve only personal decisions, there are always wider social and cultural issues at stake. For instance, while I have a personal investment in cosmetic surgery, the increasing popularity of cosmetic surgery as a solution for undesirable bodies also raises sociocultural issues much larger than my own sense of integrity. I chose to have breast implants, for example, because I did not want to go through the rest of my life flat chested, literally, since that is the outcome of bilateral mastectomies.

On the face of it, my choice appears morally respectable, and Sandy's morally frivolous, but is this really the case? I could have made other decisions. For instance, I could have chosen prosthetic breasts; I'm told there are quite good ones available. Another option was no reconstruction and no prostheses: I could have chosen simply to wear my scars as some women do, and go on with my life, sans breasts. After all, none of these options, including breast implants, carries any inherent moral weight.

My decision was based on my sense of myself, both interiorly and exteriorly. In the end I simply felt more like myself with breasts than without them. I did not feel that my moral integrity hinged upon any decision I might make, but I was consciously motivated by a desire to continue feeling "whole." I wanted to be entirely myself, interiorly and exteriorly.

Conclusion

If integrity is ultimately about one's deepest sense of wholeness, of being true to form while continuing to move on a trajectory toward the One

beyond the many, then having breast implants is consistent with my embodied integrity. Thus my integrity does not *depend* on the kind of body I
have, but neither can it be viewed entirely *apart* from my body-as-woman.
When I am entirely myself, that is, standing in a place of integrity, I know
two things with respect to my cosmetic surgery decision: (1) that reconstructed breasts do not a person make—my integrity does not hinge on
my having them, and (2) that I feel better having them. The reality is that I
have a disease that threatened my life. Choosing reconstruction was for me
a choice to continue to live widely, to live generously, to live life as wholly
as I know how. It is a decision that seems thoroughly consistent with my
own sense of self.

I suspect Sandy would make a similar claim for herself: getting breast
implants helped her feel more whole. Yet it does seem to be true that people
feel sympathy for someone who "loses" her breasts, whereas they are dis-
approving of someone else who chooses to enlarge breasts she already has.
This contrast on a personal issue gets at the underlying, or perhaps overarching, social issue that bedevils this discussion on integrity in bioethics. I
think we should consciously and vociferously lament that women grow up
in a culture where we learn to care what kind of breasts we have by mea-
suring our own bodies against cultural standards of beauty. The discussion
of breast augmentation/reconstruction is merely illustrative of the way that
we women participate in creating, affirming, and maintaining a cultural
norm that itself undermines our integrity, our wholeness. On the one hand,
I would say that women should hold fast and resist collaborating in this
cultural charade; on the other hand, I think it is really men who need to
become conscious of what these standards are doing to women, and men
who love women should protest on our behalf.

It should begin with our children. Sixteen-year-old Caitlin—and all our
nieces and sisters and friends—need to grow up in a culture that prizes
difference, not conformity. She needs to know that no matter what kind
of body she has, it is her special body that houses her beautiful self. She
needs to know that the most important thing she can develop is a sense of
integrity—that she is whole and that her body is the outward manifestation
of interior wholeness. I and her mother, and all of the women who love her,
need to model for her how to develop integrity, because it happens from the
inside out. It starts by paying attention to "that still, small voice" (1 Kings
19:11) inside, the voice of the One beyond the many that says to each of us,
"I set before you life and death; choose life" (Deuteronomy 30:19).

When we model for Caitlin and all our nieces and sisters that integrity means consistently being true to form, affirming gratitude for what is, rather than cultivating envy for what someone else has, then perhaps technologies of enhancement will hold less allure. In fairness, it must be admitted that purchasing surgery to sculpt the body from undesirable to desirable can result in increased confidence, and perhaps even happiness. What surgical enhancements cannot give us, however, is that deep sense of integrity of a self at once inviolable and simultaneously "in touch" with a wider creation, a creation both suffering and celebrating.

NOTES

This chapter is dedicated to my mother, Mary Louis Keenan, whose life illustrates what I mean more clearly than I am able to put into words. I thank Elaine Prevallet, S.L., for thinking with me and for sharing her considerable wisdom on this and related topics. I also thank Margaret Mohrmann for invaluable help in revising this chapter. Finally, thanks to Peggy Burge, my excellent reference librarian at the University of Puget Sound.

1. A full discussion of the origin of integrity may be found in Margaret Mohrmann, "On Being True to Form," this volume.

2. Lynette Lamb, "Letter from the Editor," *New Moon Network—For Adults Who Care about Girls* 7, no. 5 (May 2000): 2.

3. Samar Farah, "More Teens Opt for Plastic Surgery," *Christian Science Monitor* 92, no. 196 (August 2000): 14, 30.

4. See H. Richard Niebuhr, *The Responsible Self: An Essay in Christian Moral Philosophy* (New York: Harper & Row Publishers, 1963), passim.

5. Ibid., 106–7.

6. Ibid., 122–23.

7. Ibid.

8. I am indebted here to Alisa Carse for reminding me of Maggie Little's exploration of a similar point in "Cosmetic Surgery: Suspect Norms and the Ethics of Complicity," in *Enhancing Human Traits: Ethical and Social Implications*, ed. Erik Parens (Washington, DC: Georgetown University Press, 1998).

9. Mohrmann, "On Being True to Form," this volume.

10. Virginia Ramey Mollenkott, *The Divine Feminine: The Biblical Imagery of God as Female* (New York: Crossroad, 1983).

11. Mohrmann, "On Being True to Form," this volume.

12. Thanks to Elaine Prevallet for this insight.

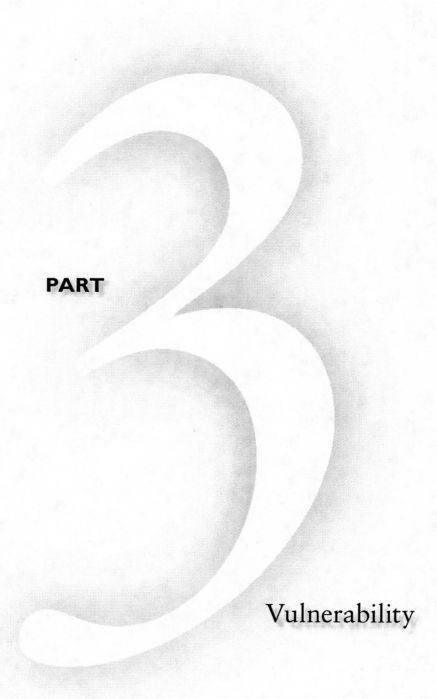

PART

3

Vulnerability

7

Vulnerability and the Meaning of Illness
Reflections on Lived Experience

S. Kay Toombs

My reflections on the vulnerability of patients and the meaning of illness have grown out of my own experience as a person living with chronic debilitating neurological disease. In 1973, at the age of twenty-nine, I was diagnosed with multiple sclerosis. Since that time I have lived with ongoing bodily disorder and increasing disability and have gained an intimate knowledge of what it means to live with chronic illness in the context of modern scientific medicine and the prevailing values of North American culture.[1]

I shall begin by exploring how predominant cultural attitudes with respect to the experience of vulnerability increase the suffering of the incurably ill. We live in a world where success is measured by the ability to shield ourselves from vulnerability, and status is marked by the degree of one's insulation from potential harm. We strive to be "financially secure," "emotionally protected," self-reliant, free from external limitation, eternally youthful. Power, wealth, professional success, celebrity, and beauty are all desired as means through which to achieve personal invincibility. At the same time, however, we sense that this struggle for invincibility and protection from harm isolates us and cuts us off from relationships. In the context of such a culture, emotional security can only be achieved through distancing oneself from others, the need for self-reliance renders dependence on others undesirable, the goals of power and wealth often demand a commitment to ruthless competition, the emphasis on such characteristics as physical "beauty" and youthfulness segregates us into different (and often opposing) social groups, and the end goal of professional "success" many times consumes our waking hours, robbing us of close family involvements. Yet, in spite of all our efforts, vulnerability inevitably intrudes into our lives. One of its most frightening forms is the experience of serious illness—a circumstance that can strike any one of us at any time without regard to worldly status or position.

In this chapter I discuss three primary manifestations of vulnerability in illness: the perception of bodily threat, the transformation of the familiar world, and the threat to personal integrity, noting how cultural attitudes regarding such things as health, independence, physical appearance, and mortality accentuate the lived experience of vulnerability and increase the patient's suffering. I then present a contrasting perspective based on my own experience for the past seven years living within a Christian community. In particular, I suggest that authentic Christian community provides an alternative cultural context founded on true relationship—a context in which it is possible for people to openly share their weaknesses and needs without fear of recrimination or condemnation from others. In this context, rather than presenting a purely negative life circumstance that is devastating to one's sense of personal wholeness, serious illness provides an opportunity to honor and serve one another and to draw closer in ever deepening relationships of selfless love. Furthermore, Christian values transform the meaning of disease, suffering, and death, thereby changing the significance of vulnerability.

Vulnerability with Respect to the Body: Body-as-Threat

At its most fundamental level, the experience of vulnerability is the perception of bodily threat. Illness breaks through our everyday complacency to remind us that we are radically dependent on (and interdependent with) our bodies.[2] That is, the lived experience of bodily breakdown is invariably accompanied by an awareness that the malfunctioning body directly threatens (or determines) one's continued physical existence. As Richard Zaner has noted, "I experience myself as implicated by my body . . . I am exposed to whatever can influence, threaten, inhibit, alter, or benefit my biological organism."[3] While it is becoming increasingly popular in sections of academe to embrace a strictly naturalistic view of human life, with no room for a discrete "mind" or "self," the fact remains that—regardless of one's philosophical viewpoint—the lived experience of bodily breakdown is invariably accompanied by an acute awareness of alienation from one's body, and as further discussion in this chapter will show, the sick person senses that the malfunctioning body directly opposes his or her personal existence in any number of ways. In other words, the illness of the physical body is inescapably *experienced* as a threat to the "self."[4] Thus, with the advent of serious illness, one feels oneself at the mercy of one's body, powerless in the face of the body's intransigence.

This perception of bodily threat represents a radical change from the way we normally relate to our bodies.[5] In health we take it for granted that our bodies will function effortlessly as we go about our daily tasks. For example, if I am seated at the breakfast table and I want a drink of orange juice, I am confident that my arm will move toward the glass and that my hand and fingers will perform the various motions required to raise the glass to my lips in order that I may drink. Indeed, I am so certain of this bodily compliance that I am barely conscious of the actual physical movement. As I reach for the glass, I am probably engaged in conversation with my husband, and I am only vaguely aware of the location of my arm. I also take it for granted that I can see the objects on the breakfast table, that I can taste the orange juice, that I can detect the smell of brewed coffee, and that I can hear my husband's voice. With respect to my mental capacities, I do not find it at all remarkable that I instantaneously recognize the difference between orange juice and coffee, that I remember where to find the breakfast items in the cupboard, or that I can carry on a detailed conversation with my spouse while performing a complex motor task that requires the coordination of intention, movement, and sensation. Under normal circumstances, I am also equally unconcerned about bodily processes such as breathing, digestion, and the beating of my heart.

Illness shatters this bodily taken-for-grantedness. The body can no longer be ignored. If some physical incapacity, such as pain, prevents me from effortlessly grasping the glass, my attention is redirected from the task at hand to the source of the difficulty—the uncomfortable sensation. In perceiving the problem to be located in my malfunctioning body, I concurrently apprehend the physicality of my body. That is, in my discomfort, I am also uncomfortably aware that my body is a material, physiological organism with its own nature—a nature that includes physiological processes, events, and structures over which I have, at best, only limited control.

This acute awareness of the physical nature of the body is accompanied by a sense of dread. I not only "have" an illness, it also "has" me. I feel myself to be at the mercy of my body, captive to physiological processes that, whether *I* like it or not, have the potential to disrupt my life. Thus, illness engenders a profound sense of bodily alienation. One experiences one's body as being an obstacle that must be overcome if one is to carry out one's projects in the world. Furthermore, not only is the body uncooperative, it is fundamentally untrustworthy.

This sense of bodily alienation is increased in the clinical encounter where the physical nature of the body is of paramount importance. The search for the cause of the disorder necessarily focuses on the body as a neuro-physiological organism. Moreover, physical signs and physiological processes are further translated into objective, quantified data (lab values, images, graphs, numbers, and so forth), all of which point to or signify some pathology "within." This focus on the innermost workings of the body increases the patient's sense that the body is a physical entity over which he or she has little or no control. In the course of clinical investigation, one comes face-to-face with the fact that most of the events and processes that take place within one's body do so without one's direct knowledge and apprehension. I do not, for example, experience the intricate workings of my heart, circulatory system, spleen, and so forth. Nor do I directly experience the degenerative process that results in the inflammation of a joint or the demyelination of my central nervous system that paralyzes my legs. Even if I have some theoretical knowledge of anatomy and physiology, the inner workings of *my own* body remain essentially beyond my ken—unfelt, unseen, unstoppable. What I grasp in this moment is my radical dependence on this vastly complex physiological system, the utter fragility of *my* physical existence and the intricate balance that is necessary to sustain *my own* physical and mental integrity.

At its deepest level the bodily threat to the self is the threat of death. In recognizing my radical dependence on my body, I sense in a terrifying way the reality of what it means to be a human being—that I am inevitably destined to die. This acute awareness of one's own finitude is not limited to those instances in which one faces life-threatening disease. Rather, any bodily breakdown shatters the illusion of invulnerability. Having once experienced illness, one recognizes that one can no longer take the body's future compliance completely for granted. This consciousness of one's own mortality is particularly frightening in the context of cultural attitudes that, to a large extent, seek to downplay or deny the inevitability of illness, suffering, and death.

Illness also forces me to recognize that I am radically dependent on my body in another way. In preventing me from performing my normal activities, the malfunctioning body reminds me that all my involvements in the world are dependent on physical and mental capacities. I can carry out my projects *only with* a certain degree of bodily compliance. For example, if I am to climb the stairs to my bedroom, it is absolutely necessary that my legs function in a particular way; if I am to hug my child, I must be able to make certain movements with my arms; if I am to work on a professional project, I must be able to concentrate (free from pain, excessive fatigue, or limitations to my mental functioning). I am not free to do as *I* will. I am only free to do what the body permits. Thus illness engenders a global threat to one's sense of self-integrity. The body is capable of inflicting not only physical harm. Given its potential to disrupt all one's plans and projects, bodily disorder also threatens to rob one of autonomy, independence, dignity, and personal integrity.

Sustained Bodily Threat—The Experience of Chronic Illness

In acute illness the sense of bodily threat is, for the most part, temporary. Once bodily function returns to "normal," one is little inclined to pay attention to the inherent fragility of the body. In the case of chronic illness, however, patients live in the presence of sustained bodily threat, uncomfortably aware that the body can never be wholly taken for granted. Ongoing physical disorder demands explicit attention. On a daily basis one must inevitably take into account specific bodily limitations that determine whether (and to what extent) one can carry out professional projects, social engagements, and family responsibilities. One can do something *only if* the body permits it. In managing chronic illness, patients must also overtly attend to the body's deficiencies in terms of taking medications, following treatment plans, and so forth, in the effort to "fend off" future threats to well-being. Even when there are lengthy periods of remission, the chronically ill remain uneasily attuned to the way the body feels and moves—always "on guard" for signs of an impending recurrence.

Paradoxically, in our society, advances in scientific medicine exacerbate the sense of bodily threat in chronic illness. Given the undeniable successes of modern technological medicine, many of us harbor unrealistic expectations about the power of medicine to "fix" medical problems and to cure disease. Indeed, we have an almost "magical" faith in doctors and in the medical system. To discover that one's disease cannot be cured is to experience the most elemental loss of control.[6]

In this respect, it is important to recognize that diagnoses mean much more to patients than simply the identification of a particular disease state. The dread diseases—such as cancer, AIDS, amyotrophic lateral sclerosis (ALS), Parkinson's, multiple sclerosis (MS), Alzheimer's—carry with them symbolic meanings that portend particularly virulent forms of threat (death, disfigurement, disability, unbearable pain, loss of independence, loss of dignity, loss of personhood). In receiving such a diagnosis, one is forced not only to deal with present physical symptoms but also to confront the personal and cultural meanings associated with the disorder. The perception of *future* threat often shapes the patient's *present* experience of illness. For instance, a study at a large MS clinic at the University of Western Ontario revealed that simply receiving a diagnosis of MS was equivalent to "moderate disability," regardless of actual physical incapacity.[7] For some people the dread of future incapacity is so disturbing that it is personally unendurable. Thus, Janet Adkins—the first person to kill herself under the direction of Jack Kevorkian—chose to end her life, while in the earliest stages of Alzheimer's, well before she actually experienced the symptoms she most feared.

Vulnerability within the World: World as Threat

In disrupting the ability to carry out everyday activities, illness transforms the character of the familiar world. In particular, the environment is experienced as overtly obstructive and unwelcoming. For example, if one is forced to use crutches, one is acutely aware of the problematic character of surrounding space. One can negotiate formerly taken-for-granted objects, such as stairs, only with the greatest of difficulty. Features of the environment (such as throw rugs or uneven walkways) actively impede one's ability to make one's way about the world. Similarly, with bodily incapacity, one experiences the obdurate nature of everyday objects. If one suffers from muscle weakness or a tremor, a favorite cooking pot presents itself as something that resists when one tries to lift it with one hand; a cup of coffee represents an acute problem—how does one bring it to one's lips without spilling the contents? These simple examples illustrate that the disruptive world is also experienced as potentially harmful. The spilled coffee can burn; a trip on the stairs can result in an injurious fall. Such experiences can also cause emotional harm in the form of embarrassment, frustration, and feelings of helplessness.

In illness, the subjective experience of space also changes in that dimensions such as near/far, high/low are intimately related to one's bodily capacities and limitations.[8] If one is sick in bed, the bathroom, which was formerly regarded as "near," may now be experienced as wearyingly "far" away. If one is in a wheelchair, the location of the light switch seems frustratingly "high," almost beyond one's reach. The physically constructed world also presents active barriers, especially for those with mobility problems. It is not only the natural terrain that may appear restrictive (distances too far to walk, slopes too steep to climb); we live in a world that has been largely designed for people with working legs. Thus, many doorways are too narrow for wheelchair users, curbs are too high to negotiate, entrances to buildings are blocked by steps. Such physical barriers also exist in the clinical context. For instance, a survey in the United States showed that women with severe disabilities are less likely to receive annual pelvic exams than able-bodied women, and 23 percent of women with spinal cord injuries reported that it was impossible to have a mammogram, either because the equipment could not be positioned for them or because there was no accessible room for mammograms.[9]

As these examples illustrate, bodily disorder changes the tenor of the familiar world. For a person with MS, the heat of summer no longer presents the inviting promise of a fun-filled day in the sun but rather the disconcerting likelihood of an increase in the severity of symptoms; for a person on crutches, the first fall of snow or a "refreshing" spring shower portends the hazard of dangerously slippery sidewalks. An illustration from my own experience demonstrates this transformation in the meaning of surrounding space. One day I was crossing the plaza outside the university library when my motorized wheelchair stopped dead in its tracks. I was surrounded by a sea of concrete embedded with decorative pebbles, marooned in the middle of a flat, completely open area with no trees, no lampposts, no benches anywhere within reach. There was no one in sight. The nearest "object" was the building, but it was absolutely impossible for me to reach it, because I can neither walk nor crawl. The space of the plaza, which a moment before had been bright, sunny, inviting, now suddenly appeared deserted and ominous. In an instant, I recognized the magnitude of my limitations and my radical dependence on technology.

For patients who require assistive devices for everyday living, dependence on technology adds another dimension to the experience of vulnerability. One is uneasily aware that mechanical breakdown can disrupt one's capacity to negotiate the world with a semblance of "normality." When the stair lift in my house malfunctioned, I was absolutely unable to reach the second floor (where the kitchen and dining room are located) for a period of weeks; when the lift on my handicap equipped van broke, I was unable to drive myself to town (to run errands, to visit friends, to get to the university); on those days when the elevator at work failed, I could not get up to the third-floor philosophy department to teach my class (or, alternatively, I was "stranded" on the third floor, unable to leave the building until a repairman appeared).

People who require assistive technology are vulnerable in another respect: the cost of such technology is exorbitant, making it impossible for many to have access to devices that could greatly improve their quality of life. Had I not possessed the financial resources to purchase a van with a wheelchair lift and hand controls, as well as a motorized wheelchair—and to build a ramp providing me access into and out of my house—I would not have been able to continue to teach at the university. (Obviously, my financial situation to a large extent depended on my ability to work, so it is a vicious circle.) None of these modifications or devices could be classified as luxurious or unnecessary. Without them, I would be unable to live a relatively independent life. Those less fortunate find themselves unable to work, unable to leave the house, unable to care for themselves, and largely "imprisoned" by their recalcitrant bodies.

Vulnerability and Personhood: The Threat to Personal Integrity

As preceding sections have shown, illness is experienced as more than simply a physiological breakdown. In disrupting daily activities and thwarting plans and projects, bodily disorder directly threatens personal integrity. In particular, patients find it difficult to retain a sense of self-worth in the face of cultural attitudes that place inordinate value on unrealistic ideals of autonomy, independence, productivity, health, and beauty and that view illness, suffering, and death as meaningless affronts to human dignity.

The perceived threat to the self at its deepest and most profound level is, of course, the existential threat of nonbeing. However, the threat to personal integrity is also intimately related to the loss of autonomy. Illness always affects the capacity to be self-reliant, to act on one's own behalf. One must inevitably depend on others to do what one has formerly been able to do for oneself. At the same time, societal values that stress the importance of self-reliance make it difficult to request and accept assistance from others. There is a strong cultural message that we should be able to look after ourselves, make our own decisions, and "stand on our own two feet." Dependence on others is perceived as weakness. In needing to ask for help, the sick person feels concretely diminished. Furthermore, connected to the cultural ideal of autonomy is the sense that each person should be able "to do their own thing" without a sense of limits. Thus, when we have to ask for help, we feel ashamed and presume we are a burden on others.

When society places inordinate value on independence and self-determination, the act of serving another is often negatively equated with self-denial. In this context, full-time caregiving is deemed less valuable than pursuing activities that will bring a state of individual fulfillment (measured in terms of professional and economic markers that signify "success" according to societal values). When caregiving is conceived of in these terms, this inevitably arouses feelings of resentment on the part of the caregiver and incalculable feelings of guilt and self-recrimination on the part of the person receiving care. Thus, in our culture, those with debilitating illness sense they expect too much of others, elderly parents constantly worry that they will end up being a burden to their children who "have their own lives to live," and there is a widespread presumption that persons with disabilities are a drain on the lives of their able-bodied partners.[10]

Given this cultural perspective, it is not surprising that the fear of "being a burden to others" can be overwhelming for patients with incurable illnesses. In 2000, 63 percent of those whose suicides were reported under the Oregon Death with Dignity Act said they feared becoming a burden to their families, friends, and caregivers. Each year this concern has been listed as an important factor in the decision to request physician-assisted suicide.[11] As Richard Zaner notes, with respect to Janet Adkins, "it was not for her [own] sake (pain, abandonment threatening to flag her resolve to be brave, and such), but for the sake of her husband, children, friends. She simply could not put them through all that."[12]

The loss of autonomy is also profoundly threatening in light of the cultural emphasis on "doing" as opposed to "being." A person's worth is judged according to his or her capacity to produce (to be useful) or to achieve a certain professional status. When we say to our children, "You can *be* whatever you want to be," what we mean is "You can achieve worth through *doing*." A person who is unable "to do" feels diminished by the inability to continue projects that are meaningful according to societal standards. Furthermore, bodily disorder necessarily disrupts social roles— wife, father, friend, homemaker—causing the sick person to feel that he or she is failing to fully contribute in areas of family and social life. In the case of acute illness, the disruption of role is temporary and therefore legitimized by others. One is excused from the usual demands of work and family life on the grounds that one will resume these responsibilities as soon as possible. If illness is ongoing, however, the inability to fully resume one's taken-for-granted roles inevitably causes one to feel diminished in person, as well as in body.

Cultural attitudes with respect to "health" (wholeness) also make it hard for chronically ill patients to accept the limitations of illness. In our society we equate "health" with the complete absence of disease and freedom from *any* physical or mental limitation. Moreover, certain ideal standards of beauty, physique, physical strength, fitness, and vigor are also often subsumed into this cultural concept of "health." Given this focus, we spend inordinate amounts of money, time, and effort in the pursuit of an illusory state of perfect physical "wholeness"—a state that is valued not so much as a means but as an end in itself. While it is obviously beneficial to seek to maintain an optimal level of physical fitness and, where possible, to avoid illness, the cultural perspective on "health" makes it difficult, if not impossible, for people to accept the reality that sickness, aging, and death are unavoidable aspects of being human. In the context of such a culture, incurable illness is an affront—an unnatural and unacceptable state of brokenness—a view that increases the patient's experience of vulnerability. The cultural perspective on "health" also makes it extraordinarily difficult for people with disabling or disfiguring conditions to retain a sense of dignity and self-worth. Because the concept of "health" includes unrealistic ideals of "beauty" and physical fitness, those who do not meet these ideals are inevitably devalued. In the eyes of the "able-bodied," there is the clear assumption that disability is incompatible with living a meaningful life.[13]

Carol Gill, a trained researcher and clinical psychologist who, for more than twenty years, has researched what it means to live with a disability notes that in a society that often believes people are better off dead than disabled the available research on suicide and disability paints a disturbing picture. She says, "it boils down to the concept of burden: We are made to feel like burdens, physically, emotionally—and that's an untenable self-view. You can't keep thinking of yourself as a burden and thrive."[14]

I can relate to Gill's observations from my own experience. When strangers observe that I am in a wheelchair, they make the immediate assumption that my situation is an essentially negative one, that I am unable to engage in professional activities and that I am wholly dependent on others. On many occasions people have said to me, "Aren't you *lucky* to have your husband!" This statement is not so much a comment on my husband's character as it is a perception that my relationship with him is wholly one of burdensome dependence. Furthermore, people overtly treat me as dependent. They invariably address remarks to my companion and refer to me in the third person, "Would *she* like us to move this chair?" This response from others is not limited to those of us who use wheelchairs. In speaking of his experience of blindness, John Hull records that people talk about him, as if he is not there: "Will you put John in the back (of the car) with you?" "No, I'll put him in the front with me."[15] Such attitudes also exist in the clinical context. In a national survey, women with severe disabilities reported that, if another person accompanied them, the doctor addressed questions to their companion, rather than speaking to them directly.[16] "Is *she* experiencing any pain?" "*She* needs to go down to the lab and get a blood test." Such common responses from others are demeaning and inevitably reinforce the disabled person's sense that disability reduces social and personal worth.

Patients also find it hard to retain a sense of self-worth in the face of other types of bodily disorder that are socially unacceptable. For many, the loss of bowel and bladder control represents the most grievous experience of loss of dignity. I can personally attest to the powerful feelings of degradation that these particular disorders can arouse. Not only is it the case that one feels reduced to the status of an infant (with the accompanying sense that, as an adult, one really "ought" to be able to exercise control) but there is the ever-present threat of public humiliation. This threat can be overwhelming in the face of cultural attitudes that treat such disorders with contempt. The possibility of public disgrace is so harrowing that many patients withdraw from social interaction. Some decide to end their lives on the grounds that incontinence robs them of all personal dignity.[17] Indeed, losing control of bodily functions is one of the three most commonly mentioned reasons for requesting physician-assisted suicide.[18]

No discussion regarding the threat to personal integrity would be complete without mentioning disorders, such as Alzheimer's and other dementias, that seem to threaten one's very identity. "The idea of losing my mind . . . losing my what I *am*," says Zaner, "is as terrifying as it is awesome. For what is ultimately threatened is my very own sense of self, not only my 'what' but my 'who.'"[19] Zaner quotes Robert Terry, a physician specializing in caring for those with Alzheimer's, who says that the real affliction of the disease is that it strips away "your very humanity, your intellect, your personality, your personal habits of hygiene."[20] While Zaner does not agree with Terry's assumption that dementia strips individuals of their humanity, and while there is much philosophical debate about the moral status of such patients, it must be stressed that, in contemporary society, many people *do* think less of the demented.[21] There is a widespread assumption that such patients are no longer fully "persons," that, in light of such affliction, family and friends have—in some sense—already "lost" the person they once loved. Thus, in these circumstances, a social "death" precedes the actual physical death. Often family members and others withdraw in the face of this perceived loss of personhood, leaving demented patients to end their days in institutional care. For Janet Adkins (and presumably also for her family) the expectation of this slide into oblivion was so demeaning that committing suicide alone in the back of a rusty old Volkswagen van seemed a preferable alternative.

Embracing Vulnerability: Reflections on Lived Experience in a Christian Community

My reflections on the vulnerability of patients and the meaning of illness have grown out of my personal experience of neurological disease in the context of prevailing cultural values. I would now like to share how becoming a Christian seven years ago broadened and transformed my understanding of these issues. In particular, I suggest that authentic Christian community may offer an alternative culture with a radically different value system—one that changes the meaning of vulnerability and enhances personal integrity.[22]

As I have noted earlier, in the wider cultural context, an important goal is to shield ourselves from all forms of vulnerability and to insulate ourselves from harm—a goal that necessarily isolates us from one another and makes it impossible to develop deep relationships based on mutual

trust. This is the case because it is precisely the willingness to open ourselves up to the possibility of hurt (to expose ourselves to vulnerability)
that allows us to enter into true relationships with other human beings.
Furthermore, the cultural perspective that places inordinate value on the
achievement of personal invincibility makes it particularly hard to accept,
and respond positively to, the inescapable vulnerability that occurs with
illness. As patients, we find it difficult to admit our needs to ourselves and
to others and to surrender our carefully nurtured attributes of self-reliance,
self-sufficiency, self-containment, and personal privacy. On the other hand,
when we are healthy, the sick remind us of our own vulnerability to illness
and disease—an uncomfortable fact that causes us to withdraw or distance
ourselves from the incurably ill and disabled. This response deepens the
chasm between caregivers and those who need care, further isolating us
from one another and deepening the sick person's sense that illness diminishes social and personal worth.

Living in a nondenominational Christian community[23] has taught me
that the desire to shield ourselves from vulnerability is not a goal to which
we should strive. As Christians, we are called to live out our lives in relationship: relationship with God and with each other. This pattern of Christian
community life provides the context in which it is both possible and necessary to embrace vulnerability—both in terms of openly acknowledging that
we have a profound need for God and in the commitment to make ourselves
transparent in our relationships with others. Because we seek to exemplify
Christian ideals that eschew selfish ambition, envy, and worldly success in
favor of love, humility, and service to others, our lives in community are
built upon a foundation of trust that enables us to share our vulnerabilities
and needs without fear of recrimination or condemnation from others. As
a result, the vulnerability that accompanies the reductions of illness is less
a purely negative life circumstance than an opportunity to share in the
miracle of relationship and the giving and receiving of the gift of selfless
love. Indeed, in imitating the example of Jesus, the suffering servant, we are
called to continually lay down our lives for one another: "Greater love has
no one than this, that one lay down his life for his friends."[24] Because love
is the cardinal value, caregiving (care of and for another) is not considered
a negative form of self-sacrifice, but rather, it is the foundation of Christian community. Far from depriving the individual, such service becomes a
means of developing the highest moral qualities of character.

The context of Christian community permits us to live out this ethic
of selfless love in very concrete ways. As an example, let me describe the

care of Robert, a forty-nine-year-old father of five who recently died from a brain tumor. During the last months of his life, friends in the community prepared meals every day for his family (when they delivered the food, they took *their* families with them, so that both families could eat and spend time together); took his children to music lessons, dentist's appointments, and to play with friends; and assisted his wife with home schooling and grocery shopping. Others took two-hour shifts to provide him with round-the-clock care (and to permit his family to attend church meetings and other events); three close friends attended to his personal needs (bathing, shaving, and so on). Others participated in a prayer chain from midnight to 6:00 A.M., seven days a week, to supplement the church's existing prayer chain for the sick. Also, as a token of love and respect, several are now tithing monetary offerings to cover the surviving family's financial needs. Such acts of service benefit not only the one who is sick. Throughout his illness, and in his dying, Robert continued to minister, not only to those who came under his pastoral care but to his caregivers and to all who came into contact with him. Indeed, dozens of young people in our community have testified that Robert's experience of grace and fortitude throughout these most difficult of circumstances has been a major influence for good in their lives.

Another example of concrete service relates to the care of a person afflicted with Alzheimer's. When the mother of a member of our fellowship developed symptoms of the disease, he brought her to live in the community, where she spent the last three and a half years of her life. To accommodate her needs, members of the fellowship built an addition onto the house that was fully equipped for wheelchair access. (These renovations were completed in a two-week period, so that she could be moved before her allotted time in the hospital expired.) To assist the family in managing her long-term care, two ladies moved in with her and took care of meals, bathing, and "entertaining." They took "Grandmommy" fishing, to the zoo, to look up long-lost relatives, out to dinner, to get ice cream, or even out for French fries and a Coke when she requested it. Grandmommy was also included in family occasions such as birthday parties, holidays, and reunions. For as long as her health permitted, she attended social activities in the community and frequently attended church services. When she became housebound, friends visited her in her home, others came to read to her, and young people came to sing. One of our craftsmen made her a cane; another fashioned a headboard for her hospital bed, as she was terrified of beds with rails; a ninety-one-year-old lady, who suffered from macular degeneration, knitted her a blanket; others sewed her "hospital gowns." When she needed round-the-clock care, several ladies volunteered to spend nights with her to relieve the primary caregivers. When Grandmommy died, she was surrounded by her family and friends. Even in the face of her loss of faculties, this atmosphere of love and care provided a healing environment that transmuted Grandmommy's extreme vulnerability into a positive circumstance through which she was able to open her heart to receiving—and even giving—love in ways that were impossible before her illness.

A central tenet of Christianity is that all human beings have intrinsic worth, regardless of any contingent circumstances. Because personal worth is independent of worldly criteria, it is not related to material success, physical or mental condition, or the individual's ability to produce. Consequently, Christian values turn upside-down the cultural perspective on the importance of "doing" versus "being." The emphasis for the Christian is not so much "How do I define myself by my role?" but "How do I live out whatever role God has provided for me? What kind of a person am I?" Believers are called to be imitators of Christ.[25] Christian virtues have to do with character. As we put on the new self and discard the values of the old,[26] we remember that Jesus said blessed are the "poor in spirit," "the meek," those who "hunger and thirst for righteousness," the "merciful," the "pure in heart."[27] We are urged to clothe ourselves with compassion, kindness, humility, gentleness, and patience, not to be envious, boastful, self-seeking, or proud.[28] While these virtues are exercised through acts, they relate to a way of being in the world that is not dependent on physical attributes or abilities and that does not look to the world's criteria of success.

When I think of the value of "being," I remember Perry, a member of our community who died from ALS at the age of thirty-five. Toward the end of his life, Perry could "do" nothing. Yet he was (and remains) a powerful influence in the lives of everyone in our community. Steadfast in faith, intelligent, thoughtful, funny, and full of joy, he was a loving father and husband who instilled lifelong values in his children. His struggles and victories in adversity encouraged all of us to persevere in our own trials. Perry did not meet the worldly ideals of beauty and strength. One day a saleswoman, eyeing his physical condition, said to his wife, "I can't believe you've stuck with him!" Yet the scriptures call us to a different standard of beauty: one that is inner rather than outer. Even the Messiah Himself was described as having "no form nor comeliness . . . and no beauty that we should desire him."[29] In judging Perry's worth solely on the basis of outward appearance, this woman completely missed his inner fortitude. Because we are so dependent on visual perception, we all find it difficult to look beyond the physical manifestation of radical disfigurement or disability. Yet unless we do, we may well miss a beautiful spiritual demeanor.

Even severe mental affliction cannot negate personal worth. Those who are afflicted with dementias are unique human beings (mother, grandmother, brother, husband) who remain inherently worthy of respect. As David Smith notes, "Although we should not treat [demented persons] as if they were not demented, we also should not pretend that they are no longer part of our family or community."[30] The values that undergird Christian community life provide a context in which the commitment to provide for the needs of such patients is a given. As Christians, we believe that patients like Grandmommy are human beings, created in the image of God, who are caught in the throes of a terrible and difficult affliction and who need all the love and care that we ourselves would want. Furthermore, because the community responds to these needs as a *body*, many members of the community are available to share in the complex provision of care.

As Christians, we are reminded that cultural attitudes that stress personal control and the postponement of death are, in fact, illusions. In recognizing that man is "but a breath," his days are like a "fleeting shadow," we comprehend the undeniable fact that there are certain givens in our lives.[31] We live always with the fragility of mortality. It is often hard for us to relinquish control in *all* areas of our lives—especially as these relate to our perception of what it means to be, say, a wife, a mother, or a breadwinner. When a dear friend became debilitated with cancer, she found it particularly hard to give up full responsibility for taking care of her own home. Yet she found that the act of relinquishing control in *that* area of her life, of submitting to her vulnerability and need, gave her the opportunity to experience depths of affection and thanksgiving that she had never felt before. If those of us who need help can come to recognize that our need is a form of communion with others (rather than a burdensome obligation that we are imposing on them), we can avoid the self-recrimination and guilt that poisons the gift of love. And if we are not willing to receive, we prevent someone from giving.

In a culture that views health and happiness as a personal right, suffering is an affront. Consequently, people tend to withdraw from the incurably ill. This enforced isolation contributes to the person's sense that he or she has become less worthy of regard. From a Christian perspective, the meaning of suffering is very different: disease, pain, discomfort, and death are understood to be very much a part of what it means to be human. Thus, in my suffering, I do not feel set apart from others, quarantined (as it were) from the rest of the human race. Furthermore, I do not feel isolated because, as a Christian, I know I serve a God who shared in the experience of suffering, a God who was "despised and rejected by men, a man of sorrows, and *familiar with suffering*" or, as the King James translation has it, "a man acquainted with grief."[32] I am comforted in the knowledge that I am never expected to face suffering alone. The God of love is Immanuel (God with Us).[33] Nor am I alone in the very real sense that I am part of the Body of Christ. In living in a close relationship with a community of believers who follow the way of the cross, of Christ's suffering, I do not face trials alone.

Becoming a Christian has also reminded me that my knowledge is necessarily fragmentary, that I can never see the "whole" picture or plan for my life.[34] Indeed, the hardest truth and a profound mystery is that, along with pain, suffering, frustration, and loss, my illness has brought with it a unique opportunity to share the meaning of illness with doctors, nurses, medical students, and other caregivers. In my writing, speaking, and teaching, I have found a life's work that has been very meaningful.

This comment is not intended to deny that human lives are often beset with unfathomable tragedy. Christianity does not turn its face away from the agony of personal suffering. Central to its message is the stark reality of the cross. When I am tempted to despair, I am reminded of the Garden of Gethsemane, of the One in whom there was no sin, but who died on the cross for my transgressions. The gospels record that in His agony, Jesus prayed until "His sweat was like drops of blood falling to the ground," asking, "My Father, if it is possible, may this cup be taken from me." But He finished his prayer with the words, "Yet not *my* will, but *Thine*."[35] In those moments when it seems impossible to pray this prayer, I think of the apostle Paul, who prayed three times that the "thorn in his flesh" would be taken away, only to receive the promise, "My grace is sufficient for you, for my power is made perfect in weakness."[36]

The reality of the cross is at odds with the cultural emphasis on autonomy. In imitating Christ, believers are called to relinquish absolute control over their lives. Jesus' admonition is to "pick up your cross and follow Me," every single day.[37] Along the way, we may well have to face the burdens of illness, suffering, and disability, and inevitably we will experience the reductions of aging and death. These reductions do not diminish one's intrinsic worth as a human being. Furthermore, if I am to stay true to the example given by Jesus in Gethsemane, I cannot arbitrarily circumscribe the limits of the cross I am willing to bear. The desire to "limit the cross" is motivated by the wish to escape a "worst case scenario" that seems personally unendurable. Yet, as Christians, we have found that one can experience supernatural grace even in these direst of circumstances. As she neared death, our dear friend Helen shared, "The *one thing* I don't want to happen is to feel that I'm suffocating." On the night she died, her worst fears were realized when she began to struggle for breath. Yet, as she gave herself to the prayer "Not *my* will but *Thine*," she almost instantly experienced an overwhelming sense of peace. "I keep thinking of that song, 'God has been so good to me. Forever I will praise His name,'" she said. Then she smiled, whispered, "I love you," closed her eyes, and died.

As Christians, we believe that the cross is not the end of the story in God's eternal purposes. Our faith calls us to look beyond the present suffering to a future glory that will be revealed to us if we are willing to stay the course. It also assures us that nothing—"tribulation, distress, persecution, famine, nakedness, peril or sword" nor "death, nor life, nor angels, nor principalities, nor powers, nor things present, nor things to come"—shall be able to separate us from the love of God.[38] We are encouraged, therefore, to persevere in the face of trials, trusting in God and knowing that beyond the agony of Calvary lies the promise of the empty tomb. This promise is no illusion. We have a "cloud of witnesses"[39] who have gone before us and who have testified to its truth. I have space to share only one of many testimonies: at the time of his death, due to the ravages of ALS, Perry had been unable to talk for more than a year. He regained the ability to speak just moments before he died. In a clearly discernible voice, he used his dying breaths to tell those gathered with him to share with everybody that God would remain "faithful *all the way to the end*" in each of their lives too.

From an immanent perspective, perseverance in the face of suffering is meaningless. From an eternal perspective, there is a larger wisdom that places disease, suffering, and death within the context of a cosmic narrative of the power of love overcoming even the power of death. Indeed, in this context, the willingness to surrender to our personal vulnerability, to humble ourselves by exposing our manifold weaknesses to others, is the avenue that opens us up to the miracle of relationship—a miracle that brings tears of gratitude and thanksgiving even in the most difficult circumstances. Within the context of a community of individuals dedicated to opening themselves to one another without masks or defensive images, we can all draw closer in sanctified relationships. We do not fear that others will use our weakness and openness to their own advantage, but instead believe that they will open themselves up in return, as the spirit of love that exposed itself through the defenseless Lamb of God becomes so real in our lives as to conquer again and again even the final enemy, death itself.

Conclusion

In reflecting on what it means to live in a Christian community, I am reminded of the centrality of the covenantal relationship in our lives as Christians: relationship with God and with each other. This covenantal relationship is built upon the foundation stone of self-sacrificial love—a love that is exemplified in the life and death of Jesus and that finds its fullest expression in the context of a body of believers, the Body of Christ. The values and practices that spring from this foundation of self-sacrificial love provide a context in which it is possible to embrace vulnerability, to openly acknowledge our need for God and for one another. This acknowledgment of shared dependency and need in turn reveals the way for deep and lasting relationships that exemplify the commitment to honor and serve one another in love. This ethic of selfless love necessarily enhances personal integrity.

NOTES

1. I am thinking here of values that are prevalent in North American culture and in Western scientific medicine although, to the extent that these values have spread to other parts of the world, these comments apply to the meaning of illness in other cultures.

2. Of course, as phenomenologists have pointed out, we are *embodied* beings and therefore we are necessarily dependent on, and interdependent with, our bodies. We do not just "have" bodies, we "exist" our bodies. For a discussion on the phenomenological perspective on embodiment and its application to medicine, see S. Kay Toombs, "Introduction: Phenomenology and Medicine," in *Handbook of Phenomenology and Medicine* (Dordrecht, Neth.: Kluwer Academic Publishers, 2001), 5–10.

3. Richard M. Zaner, *The Context of Self: A Phenomenological Inquiry Using Medicine as a Clue* (Athens: Ohio University Press, 1981), 52.

4. With the rise of "evolutionary psychology" and related disciplines, there is, of course, a growing trend to nullify any distinction between mind and body and, specifically, to negate the notion of a discrete self. This view traces back, in the Western tradition, at least to Hume, who denied the reality of "our own continued

existence as persons." In his view, "When we look inside ourselves, we do not find an impression of a continuous self but only bundles of changing ideas. Every attempt to defend our belief in our personal identity falls before critical questioning." See Richard H. Popkin, ed., *Columbia History of Western Philosophy* (New York: MJF Books, 1999), 457. This view has become more widespread in modern-day thought, as expressed in a 1999 joint lecture in which Richard Dawkins asked Stephen Pinker, "Am I right to think that the feeling I have that I'm a single entity, who makes decisions, and loves and hates and has political views and things is a kind of illusion that has come about because Darwinian selection found it expedient to create that illusion of unitariness rather than let us be a society of mind?" Pinker agreed, saying that "the fact that the brain ultimately controls a body that has to be in one place at one time may impose the need for some kind of circuit . . . that coordinates the different agendas of the different parts of the brain to ensure that the whole body goes in one direction." The text of this debate, "Is Science Killing the Soul?" can be viewed at www.edge.org/3rd_culture/dawkins_pinker/debate_p1.html. According to Susan Blackmore, "We may feel as though we have a special little 'me' inside, who has sensations and consciousness, who lives my life, and makes my decisions. Yet, this does not fit with what we know about the brain." See Susan Blackmore, "Meme, Myself, I," *New Scientist* 161, no. 2177 (1999): 40–44. Without at this point discussing the philosophical and scientific problems with this hypothesis, the reality of illness, and particularly chronic illness, is that one does not experience self as an illusory entity. Since (as Blackmore herself notes) the conclusions of Dawkins, Pinker, Blackmore, and their associates seem in many ways to concur with the Buddhist tradition, according to which "the bodhisattva no longer . . . perceives *a* self, *a* being, *a* person," because he has entered into the state of nirvana, which entails "annihilation of the ego," perhaps they, in keeping with this Buddhist view, would regard these forms of vulnerability in illness, and of the attendant sense of threat to the self, as illusory. However, in talking to thousands of patients and caregivers throughout the United States, Canada, and western Europe (and in living with debilitating illness for more than thirty years), I can attest to the fact that (in these cultures at least) chronically ill patients perceive the sense of a threat to the "self" as something very real, something to be taken seriously and to be dealt with as a real, not illusory, threat. For a discussion on these Buddhist beliefs, see Douglas S. Soccio, *Archetypes of Wisdom* (Belmont, CA: Wadsworth, 1998), 320–21.

5. S. Kay Toombs, *The Meaning of Illness: A Phenomenological Account of the Different Perspectives of Physician and Patient* (Dordrecht, Neth.: Kluwer Academic Publishers, 1992), 70–75.

6. S. Kay Toombs, "Sufficient Unto the Day: A Life with Multiple Sclerosis," in *Chronic Illness: From Experience to Policy*, ed. S. K. Toombs, D. Barnard, and R. A. Carson (Bloomington: Indiana University Press, 1995), 3–23.

7. This information was given to me by Dr. George Ebers, M.D., University of Western Ontario, London, Canada, in 1992.

8. S. Kay Toombs, "Reflections on Bodily Change: The Lived Experience of Disability," in *Handbook of Phenomenology and Medicine*, ed. S. K. Toombs (Dordrecht, Neth.: Kluwer Academic Publishers, 2001), 247–61.

9. This information was given to me by Margaret Nosek, Ph.D., director of the Center for Research on Women with Disabilities, Baylor College of Medicine, Houston, Texas, based on unpublished responses to comprehensive national surveys conducted by the Center 1992–95. See also Margaret Nosek and C. A. Howland, "Breast and Cervical Cancer Screening among Women with Physical Disabilities," *Archives of Physical Medicine and Rehabilitation Supplement* 5 (1997): 39–44.

10. Albert B. Robillard, *The Meaning of a Disability: The Lived Experience of Paralysis* (Philadelphia: Temple University Press, 1988).

11. Physician-assisted suicide legislative statute and reports, 1998–2002, Oregon Department of Health Services, available at www.ohd.hr.state.or.us/chs/pas/ors.cfm (accessed February 19, 2004).

12. Richard M. Zaner, *Conversations on the Edge: Narratives of Ethics and Illness* (Washington, DC: Georgetown University Press, 2004), 85.

13. Barry Corbet, "Physician Assisted Death: Are We Asking the Right Questions?" *New Mobility* (May 2003). In 1992, the Dutch Pediatric Association issued guidelines for killing severely handicapped newborns. See "Euthanasia in the Netherlands": 4, International Task Force on Euthanasia and Assisted Suicide, available at www.internationaltaskforce.org /fctholl.htm (accessed February 18, 2004).

14. Carol Gill, quoted in Josie Byzek, "What's in Your Head? Who Put It There?" *New Mobility* (May 2004): 37–38.

15. John M. Hull, *Touching the Rock: An Experience of Blindness* (New York: Pantheon Books, 1990), 112–13.

16. Margaret Nosek, unpublished surveys, 1992–95.

17. As a personal example, a close relative tragically cited this, and the fear of becoming a burden to others, as the primary reasons for killing himself.

18. Physician-assisted suicide legislative statute and reports, Oregon Department of Health Services, 1998–2002.

19. Zaner, *Conversations on the Edge*, 78.

20. Ibid.

21. Ibid., 81.

22. Portions of this discussion on the lived experience of illness in the context of Christian community have been included in my article "Living and Dying with Dignity: Reflections on Lived Experience," *Journal of Palliative Care* 20, no. 3 (2004): 193–200. Reprinted with permission.

23. My purpose in this section of the chapter is to share my lived experience of incurable debilitating illness in the context of the practices and values of a nondenominational Christian community and to show how these particular values and practices provide an alternative perspective on the vulnerability of illness. It is not possible in the context of this chapter to provide a detailed account of the vision, roots, and cultural position of our community (nor is it the appropriate place to do so). I should perhaps explain that we draw probably the greatest portion of our beliefs and lifestyle and values from the Anabaptist tradition, although there have been additional major influences such as Pietism and others. Although I am aware that our community is unique in some respects, the core values that I describe are not unique to our small community but derive from the New Testament and,

indeed, from the Judeo-Christian tradition generally and are values that are pursued by those who seek to follow this tradition. My intent is to show how the alternative cultural core values of our community of Christians provide a context in which it is possible to open ourselves up to (and even embrace) our shared vulnerabilities and needs and to thereby experience deep and lasting relationships that exemplify the love of God and provide personal affirmation in even the direst of circumstances. Some readers of this manuscript have indicated that they would like to learn more about our community. Because space prohibits me from providing detailed information in this article, I would be happy to provide such information to anyone who cares to contact me.

24. John 15:13. The scriptural references in this section are taken from the *New American Standard Bible* (Anaheim, CA: Foundation Publications, 1995) except where a different translation is noted in the text.

25. John 13:12–15; Eph. 5:1–2.

26. Col. 3:1–17.

27. Matt 5:3–11.

28. 1 Cor. 13:1–13; Col. 3:12–15.

29. Isa. 53:2.

30. David Smith, quoted in Zaner, *Conversations on the Edge*, 84.

31. Psalm 39:4–5; 144:4; James 4:14.

32. Isa. 53:3.

33. Matt. 1:23; Isa. 7:14.

34. Prov. 3:5–6.

35. Matt. 26:39; Mark 14:33–36; Luke 22:41–44.

36. 2 Cor. 12:7–10.

37. Matt. 10:38–39, 16:24–25; Mark 8:34–35; Luke 9:23–24, 14:27.

38. Rom. 8:35, 39.

39. Heb. 12:1–2.

8

A Meditation on Vulnerability and Power

Richard M. Zaner

Hospitalized for more than four months, Mrs. Oland, who just turned seventy-two years old, has been married for many years to a gentle, caring man, Thomas Oland. Several years her senior and still in good health, Mr. Oland is looked to for making crucial decisions during those times when his wife is unable to do so. They have three adult children, two of whom live in other cities and the other in the same city as her parents. One daughter, Janice, and the son, Charlie, are regular visitors; the younger daughter (and youngest child) works and is unable to visit often; like her brother, she lives in another city; unlike him, she is able to get away from her job only infrequently.

Mrs. Oland has been found to have frequent air leaks in her lungs (recurrent pneumothoraces), respiratory failure, prolonged hypotension, and end-stage renal disease (ESRD), any one of which could rapidly become life threatening. Her attending physician at this hospital (who has not treated her before) is Dr. Stanley Langston, who wrote in her medical chart that her prognosis is "dismal." She is not expected to recover renal function or be weaned from the ventilator or the gastrointestinal (GI) tube—she is clearly terminally ill. Only sporadically alert, she is often unable to make decisions. A pulmonologist penned a note in her chart that "continued treatment is futile" and merely "prolongs dying," and he recommended a Do-Not-Resuscitate (DNR) order. However, Mr. Oland insisted that they "do everything possible"; full supports are continued.

A neurologist's note states that Mr. Oland, Janice, and Charlie are "emotionally unprepared and confused," and this prompts an ethics consult request. After a number of conversations, several themes behind Mr. Oland's reluctance to accept the DNR eventually became clear: mainly profound guilt that he had regularly refused to listen to his wife when she tried to talk about her condition and that he would never be able to now. He had shushed her any time she tried to discuss what to do when her final days came; yet both knew this would happen.

Since her hospitalization, he has been wracked with guilt and self-loathing: what neither had wanted—a terminally ill Mrs. Oland, bed-ridden and plugged into the vent and feeding tube, which only prolonged her dying—was now stark reality. In a way, this came about because no one at first seemed willing to discuss just what to do in the event of such a crisis. But their unhappy situation arose as well from flaws in communication with physicians and nurses—doubtless resulting in part from a kind of institutionalized impatience with details and a refusal or inability to address the unspoken. Still, resolution eventually occurred; she managed to die peacefully, with the family bearing up well.

An Overview of the Encounter

I was asked to consult by the attending physician. When I talked with him, he said right off that he had a "clue" for me: Mr. Oland's strained reaction each time Dr. Langston brought up the need for a feeding tube. I learned, however, that the clue indicated something quite different from what he suspected.

That difference became evident during conversations with Mr. Oland. It was not the existence of his wife's feeding tube that upset him (or his children), but rather what he took to be its real significance. Several years prior, and just after she learned about how serious her condition was, he said almost in passing, that his wife had told him about a friend who had yanked out her feeding tube—she didn't want "the damned thing," did not want her death prolonged. The story jolted him, for he *knew* his wife had to be talking about herself, and he couldn't bring himself to face that at the time. He became seriously locked into grief and guilt, which silently boiled beneath the surface.

Because she couldn't decide for herself, her doctors turned to him for a decision about limiting treatment (the DNR), and later about removal of all supports. He was stunned by the DNR and played dumb, telling them, and himself, that he couldn't answer those questions. As he came to appreciate later, he really did know his wife's wishes, but couldn't bring himself to say it—then, or even when he realized that "Myra needs me to be strong, and I've failed." Having to face the prospect of her actually "going to die," and realizing that he would soon have to witness it, was too much for him to bear.

Nevertheless, she finally managed to make herself heard when she regained temporary alertness. She remained resolute to be allowed to die with as much dignity as possible; she was also determined to rescue her husband from his suffering. She understood what was happening to him and her children. A courageous woman, she was able to help the others, Mr. Oland especially, respect her wishes and accept her death. Unlike what too often happens to such patients in what Jan van den Berg once described as our "palaces of compulsive cure,"[1] she managed to die with what seemed to me considerable dignity.

Tentative Maps

As I later tried to understand and to attempt to help these people and their caregivers, it seemed to me imperative to immerse myself deliberately[2] in this situation, starting from the moment I first walked into her room. Significantly, when I first entered, it was immediately evident that her vulnerability was the predominant phenomenon: it best characterized her condition, and her husband's as well. Here is the phenomenon as best as I can reconstruct it.

She is lying there on the bed, very still, the ventilator's soft chug the loudest sound in the room, her rising and falling chest under the light sheet her only movement. Then her eyes flicker open and shut, partially and irregularly, without apparent stimulus. When I say, "Mrs. Oland?" she turns toward me, her eyes open, but she seems unfocused; her eyes wander about, unseeing. I speak again: "Mrs. Oland? I am Dr. Zaner, from clinical ethics. Your doctor asked me to stop by to see you." She doesn't orient to or even seem to hear me (my mistake, I later learn). I say "good-by" and leave as quietly as I can, hearing a sort of "Uhng." I stop and turn around, but she seems unchanged, and I turn again and leave.

Some days later, she becomes more alert and things are markedly different. When I enter her room this time, others are there, including Dr. Langston, but she turns her head and looks at me. Despite the tubes and monitor lines snaking into her body, she is very much, in Alfred Schutz's term, a lively, vivid presence.[3] This is in bold contrast to my first visit to her room, when she seemed more an inert mass than a live bodily presence.[4] Though still physically voiceless, she now has a kind of voice: when I say my name, her eyes sparkle with recognition and obvious humor at my surprise that she knows my name. As Dr. Langston talks, she displays impatience followed by gestured understanding: of course she knows what's going on. Mention of her husband's difficulties brings tears, averted eyes, a slow raising and dropping of her hands, expressive of deep sadness and regret.

In another of Schutz's wonderful idioms, she and I are face-to-face[5] with each other: she within her still unfolding (though nearly completed) biography, me within mine.[6] Our encounter, mere promise at first, is now gradually textured with our respective biographies; although incomplete, the relationship is dense with promised anecdotes and themes embedded in stories, hers and my own, invited in every glance and gesture, however brief the moment. Each time we meet I enter her history and find her a part of my own—which I now partly relate.

"The" room is her room; entering, I move into her (temporary) domain even though I think (mistakenly) that her notice is too diffuse to support later recall. It is nevertheless perfectly obvious that she is a person, although critically ill. She is neither mere physical mass nor cadaver. Later, her gestures, frail though definite, are unmistakably those of a sick person.

Everything in her room is arranged in very specific and powerful ways with respect to her. She is the center; everything in the room is there for her—the equipment, activities, procedures. Indeed, a kind of de-centering is evident: here, in this room, "you" and "I" matter far less than she. Talk centers on her: she is the one who matters here. Not only our words but even our gestures are muted, as if our ability to wander around the room or shake hands should be kept alertly quiet—unwelcome reminders of things once within her repertoire but now no longer.

Her Vulnerability

Anyone entering this patient's hospital room can note that even though vulnerable, she displays a striking, commanding presence simply by lying on the bed. Her vulnerability is at once dramatic and imposing; it commands attention. This is in conspicuous contrast to the social and other relational imbalances due to her illness and her relationship with others, especially those charged with her care. Her relationship to them is *asymmetrical*, with power (in the form of knowledge, skills, access to resources, social legitimacy, and legal authority) on their side, not hers.[7] Her doctor professes the knowledge and skills necessary for diagnosing and treating her; she does not. He, not she, has access to resources (diagnostic technologies, equipment, prescription drugs, consultants, hospitals, etc.). Yet all these factors are designed *for her*; they are ordained for the clinical sake of the debilitated and distressed.

The illness experience is thus quite unique,[8] just as are the specific efforts to do something about her illness. Intrusive and unwanted, illness seems a capricious irruption into our ongoing lives. Marked by a sense of urgency, it is laced with underlying threats of compromise and loss—of time, ability, funds, family, and friends, ultimately ending in death. Illness in the broadest sense cuts into the fabric of social and individual life, abruptly alters usual relations with other people, and severely compromises the sense of self, others, and world.

Mrs. Oland often does not know clearly what's going on, much less what could and should be done about it; her energy is rather absorbed and focused by trauma, pain, anxiety, regret, and loss. Dr. Langston's very presence implies that he possesses some ability to help, heal, or cure; yet, most likely, she doesn't even know whether or not he can do so. Despite his, or any physician's, claims of competence and trustworthiness, she has no direct knowledge or experience that could possibly serve to warrant her initial act of putting her trust in him.[9] Like most of us, she may have tried to ignore her illness, or to rely on her own resources—a dietary regimen of vitamins, minerals, and so forth. Except for that, help from another person has to be sought, and thereby she enters into that structurally asymmetrical relationship powerfully reinforced by the institution, the hospital, itself.

The Historical Tradition

It is perfectly evident: the most prominent phenomenon here is patient vulnerability, itself underscored by the asymmetry; not merely a formality of socially instituted relationships, it is an existential, often painful reality. As one patient poignantly said, "you have to trust these people, the physicians, like you do God . . . if they don't take care of you, who's going to?"

I find an echo of an ancient enigma in these plaintive words, more sensed than known explicitly at every moment I am involved with any patient. Medical historian Ludwig Edelstein saw the essential point, reflecting on ancient medicine: "What about the patient who is putting himself and 'his all' into the hands of the physician?"[10] Is the patient's initial trust in a physician warranted? The sense of it may be difficult, even embarrassing, to admit: that there are serious temptations implicit to every relationship with a patient, at the heart of which is a sense of actual power over the existentially vulnerable patient who is open and exposed—to gazes, touches, voices, not to mention the often more intrusive "interventions" common to many medical encounters.

The puzzle lies at the heart of the physician-patient relationship and is, I think, at the core of the Hippocratic tradition. This may be best understood if we consider briefly the Hippocratic oath's mythic sources, in which we find the god Apollo and his progeny, Aesculepius, the god of healers and patients. In the very act of taking the oath, these ancient healers understood that they were thereafter pledged to help all sick and injured people, without prejudice. They understood that their "art" involved them with sick people and their families in uniquely potent and intimate ways.

The oath signified that these ancient "healers" were entrusted by the gods through a sacred vow to help afflicted people in regard to both soul and body. Consequent to the vow, the healer accepted certain fundamental responsibilities. First and foremost, it was said, the healer had to turn his attention to *himself*, to heal himself before ever trying to serve others. It also seems clear that this vow made the *vulnerability* of every patient the vital center. On the patient's side, this vulnerability, I suggest, is the root phenomenon of the moral order in this domain and is therefore marked, as Edelstein insists,[11] by a blend of *justice* and *self-restraint* on the healer's side. Accompanying both, as I see it, is the phenomenon of *courage*.

Behind this covenant is an understanding of social life, which shows a strong sense of the power inherent to the "art," its tempting potential for manipulation, influence, and even violence to the patient and family who come to be "in the hands" of a healer. Acting on behalf of the sick person and maintaining strict silence about all things learned from the relationship were as integral to the oath as were certain conducts strictly banned (giving abortifacients, assisting a suicide, doing a lithotomy).

It is precisely in view of patient vulnerability, I am convinced, that there developed an urgent demand to "cause no harm" (*nolo nocere*) unless in the service of providing benefit. The ancient healers clearly recognized how their unique position provided them ways to take advantage of people who are at their most vulnerable and open to manipulation.[12] Their oath strongly suggests a recognition of this challenge and temptation and is thus among the earliest phases of a sophisticated moral cognizance.

The Ancient Enigma

But it is just this moral cognizance that poses the searching moral issue: What could possibly prompt a healer *not* to take advantage of a vulnerable person, precisely in view of that vulnerability? There is another equally ancient and powerful myth about the temptations of having actual power, which helps to elicit this cognizance: the Gyges story in book 2 of Plato's classic study of the life of the polis, *The Republic*[13]—a scene that postulates a very different kind of social order than does the Hippocratic tradition. In Plato's scene, people pursue their own self-interest, because injustice is more powerful than justice. Even if ruled by law, compliance is always against their will—whether from fear of retribution, indolence, or simply lack of power to do as they wish. After this setting is described, Socrates tells about the fabled Gyges, a shepherd serving the king of Lydia. An earthquake opened up a deep chasm, and peering down, Gyges spied a hollow bronze horse with a human corpse beside it wearing nothing but a gold ring. He promptly climbed down, removed the ring, and placed it on his own finger. That evening he chanced to twist the ring's removable enclosing rim and promptly became invisible, without, apparently, anyone noticing. Amazed, he turned the rim the other way and presto! reappeared. His next actions are well-known: on his monthly visit to the king, he made himself invisible, seduced the queen, and with her acquiescence killed the king and took the crown for himself. This is precisely what "justice" is supposedly all about: each of us seeks to gain advantage over others; "just" and "unjust" are but social conventions, defined by those with power. Morality is thus the invention of those in power, used to enforce their wishes.

This is a dramatic example of the enigma: doesn't the Gygean version of human social life in fact tell us that, having the advantage of such power, the healer in a Gygean world *will* surely take advantage of those who are vulnerable *precisely because* they are vulnerable, open to manipulation and seduction? In such a vision of social life, the healing art is perforce little more than a sham, the Hippocratic oath merely a façade masking the exercise of power, vulnerability in truth but a motive for its use. The basis of the healer-patient relationship is the asymmetry of power in favor of the healer against the vulnerability of the patient. Although clothed in social courtesies and a bedside manner, as Hobbes later insisted in his *Leviathan*, beneath it all is the self-seeking of Gyges and the fear of others' possessing and using the ring of power.

Each myth invokes its own vision of the common world, including clinical encounters: a person with power and advantage confronts another who is at a decided disadvantage. In the Hippocratic tradition, the resulting temptations formed the basis for the oath's repeated injunctions never to take advantage of the sick person. If the Gyges tale were the corrective view of social life, any attempt to help the sick person would only make the vulnerable person less vulnerable, hence more of a threat.

Awakening a Moral Sense

Every clinical encounter in the Hippocratic tradition is haunted by the story of Gyges and its temptations to take advantage of the vulnerable person. As I noted, though, there is something peculiar, even paradoxical, about Mrs. Oland's vulnerability—and about those immediately affected, such as Mr. Oland or their adult children. It is in her vulnerability that Mrs. Oland is, nevertheless, truly *compelling*; she exercises a special, powerful attraction simply—perhaps incongruously—by lying there, bedridden and unable to help herself.[14]

For instance, walking into her room, I sense that she is a sort of center of gravity, pulling others' looks, words, and actions toward her: it is *she* who appeals for response, *she* who needs help. It seems that her very *difference* is what attracts. Her illness renders her vulnerable; over that is my health and ability to act. I find myself thinking about the dramatic contrast between her hapless gaze (diffuse, unaware), cast of brow (appeal, fear), or way of speaking (hand, head) and her daughter's expressive face (welcoming or threatening), the glow of her cheeks, her speech (irony or seriousness). Don't these characteristics of illness, the muting of aliveness, its very silence, bring it to experiential prominence for our moral regard?

To be sure, Mrs. Oland's very vulnerability left her open to the actions of other people—to medical and nursing examinations, for instance. Yet that very exposure is morally commanding and compelling. I sensed it immediately on entering her room: *Be cautious! Touch, if you must, but carefully! Watch what you say!* Note how potent is this vulnerability; it attracts, directs anyone who approaches to *be vigilant* in what is said and done. A need to be restrained yet concerned silently governs. Would it not be monstrous to take advantage of her?

The *Ec-stasis* of Moral Sensitivity

In this way, Mrs. Oland's vulnerability *evokes or solicits a moral sense.*[15] The very structural asymmetry of the relationship is, paradoxically, turned on its head, for it is precisely what brings out an elemental yet commanding sense of alertful[16] responsibility,[17] as was first appreciated by ancient Hippocratic physicians. Their firm insistence on justice and self-restraint (and courage) is striking, for the physician-patient relationship places power on the side of the physician, not the patient—even as it brings patient vulnerability to the center.

The real puzzle is just this: what, in the end, is the source of that evocation, as opposed to the quite different tradition implicit to the Gyges myth? I propose that it is precisely that existential vulnerability that, negatively expressed, awakens the responsibility *never to take advantage of* the sick or the debilitated,[18] and positively, in the terms of the Hippocratic oath, to act always *on behalf of* that individual. In both senses, this is a *moral* awakening, for at every point one faces a choice of "yes" or "no," and to act accordingly.

There is in this embodied experience a primordial pull to be *mindful* of this woman within her actual circumstances. To be mindful, in turn, heralds a sort of de-centering, an elemental *ec-stasis*—I am pulled *beyond* myself *to* her, vigilant to *her*; it may even be that I become myself in this vigilance. What and who she is, what and who I am,—that odd pronominal "self" each of us shelters, nourishes, conceals, or, infrequently, reveals— are thereby brought about and made uniquely present. "Self" in these terms is always an accomplishment that each of us is brought into; it is what is gifted to each through encountering each other within this *ec-stasis*.

This rudimentary mindfulness is drawn out of the encounter with the vulnerable other self. Moreover, in my case, this critical pull and reach beyond myself is also *invited*, even required, by the vulnerable other, and it powerfully lifts me up into a moral observance of this fragile, undemanding woman whose family is mourning and whose husband is torn up by his early refusal to discuss her death and life. Because clinical relations require at times profound intimacies such as these, they have an unavoidable and potently seductive character; the other side of her vulnerability is her tempting openness to being used, manipulated. The paradox is thus apparent:[19] her very availability to manipulation evokes my own availability to be at her disposal and thus not take advantage. In this very display of seductive possibility of taking advantage of her, whose life in the nature of the case is precarious and compellingly exposed, is a commanding voice: any of us is able take advantage *precisely because* of her vulnerability, but it is for this reason that this ought never be done.

Alfred Schutz has vividly demonstrated that, in our daily lives, for the most part we live, act, and think within a more or less thoroughly taken-for-granted context of relatively well-defined typifications (types of people, sorts of things and relations, kinds of activities). So long as our affairs remain relatively settled and unruffled, we simply expect everything to continue as it has thus far.[20] Our typical and typifying ways of thinking and acting together in the everyday world are maintained so long as nothing comes along to upset or unsettle them, "valid" for all practical purposes.

Such an unsettling of taken-for-granted expectations is at the heart of encounters between strangers, because the stranger is essentially one who has no choice but to wonder about, to question nearly everything that is taken for granted by the people approached; indeed the stranger, Schutz emphasizes, is one without a shared history.[21] The Olands and I (but also Dr. Langston and others in the hospital) were strangers in precisely this sense; only her illness brought her within our domain. What is for each of us respectively the familiar and the routine, the settled and the comfortable—including the common tongue—are now no longer able to be taken granted. Rather than proceeding on the presumption of shared values and outlooks, conversations with the stranger assume the forms of probings and explorations—and are hence always problematic and textured by uncertainties.

Conversation and Trust

Each clinical conversation is a gradual search for, and understanding of, the patient's (and family's) imperative search for what's wrong and what can be done to help, so that they can also understand (and be understood). It is often a seeking-for-another to help in that search—to share in the experience of asking and answering, talking and listening, appealing and responding. The patient's appeal thus involves the actual process of questioning, examining, challenging, doubting—to do *whatever* it takes to resolve things, to become *free from* not knowing and *free for* understanding, and ultimately, for doing the right thing.

Here, the clinical conversation is at least two-sided (and is often even more complicated): the seeking by the patient (and family), which is an appeal for response from the caregivers, and the response solicited, which must be *responsive* to the appealer's need to know—and the one responding must be *responsible* for the response given. Thus to question is to open oneself up to (or to find oneself opened up by) some other person who professes the ability to answer and, by answering, to help. It is to acknowledge a vital not knowing and need to know—thus it is to stand ready to listen to whatever responsively and responsibly speaks to that appeal. Clearly, what guides the patient as he or she sifts through possible responses to the not knowing is that the need to know is *vital*. On first admission, Mrs. Oland wants to know: How serious is it? Is this the final stage? Can I be helped? And, beneath it all, Mr. Oland wants to know vitally as well: Is this "it"?

This vital form of speaking and listening to and with the other within the asymmetric relationship, it has seemed to me, is the vital core of *dialogue*, thus the remarkable way in which narration seems so appropriate to express the clinical encounter is most suitable for "telling" what's going on. In admitting and sharing my not knowing and my need to know, I reveal and share who and what I am, and in this act I *invite* the other to do so with me—trusting that the other will not take advantage of me in my not knowing, my vulnerability.

The issue for Mr. Oland is likewise apparent: he asked for help in various ways, and at several points directed his appeal specifically to me. He desperately wanted and needed to know, even as he resisted asking and knowing; their children, too, wanted and needed to know. When Mr. Oland indicated his acceptance of my invitation to talk, his act invited a dialogue to begin. Perhaps not fully aware of what that would involve, to be sure;

the subsequent dialogue exposed him to my probing for what was really bothering him, as in turn, my own participation invited his questioning of me. Our dialogue entailed attentive listening and responding.

But is there anything that can ensure that anyone, myself in particular, will actually be responsive and responsible? That I will be drawn in to his concerns? That I will help and won't take advantage of him? Perhaps not even his urgent asking and voicing his need is enough. Even vital needs do not guarantee relevant responses.

Paradoxically, even though presenting his own sort of vulnerability, with the balance of power on the side of the providers, myself included, Mr. Oland yet was the only one who could be responsible for initiating subsequent talk (perhaps solely by *letting* it happen); had he not made his need plain, none of us could rightly try and respond. But when he did agree to talk, his questions were obviously genuine; the problem was that he could not be assured beforehand that my response would also be genuine, as that was what he wanted and needed. Response cannot be guaranteed despite the quality of the appeal: Isn't this the pathos of every moral concern when we seek to share it with others?

Dialogue and Violence

Clearly, the nature of the temptation from Gyges, which remains very much with us, cautions that we not be naïve, especially where patients and families, doctors and others in health care, are involved. Still, given the dialectics of vulnerability and power—the necessary asymmetry of helping—is there a way to avoid coercion, manipulation, and violence, thus taking advantage of those who are least able to resist? If we must be constantly on the alert for violence by others—the core concern in Hobbes's *Leviathan*—is dialogue even possible? This is a troubling issue, especially when grappling with ethical issues in clinical medicine: it is in this way that Gyges still haunts the clinical world.

In short, can any of the well-known tricks and deceptions, even the ironies so deeply entrenched in our relationships with each other, be avoided and there still be dialogical discourse? It may be that, perhaps paradoxically, the one who initiates the dialogue must at the same time be a sort of *reminder*, precisely through openly presenting himself or herself as vulnerable and ignorant—a reminder that the other is and must be free to respond or not, to deceive or not, to refuse, like many of the Socratic interlocutors, even to engage with the questioner. Yet, while I am inclined to remind the vulnerable person that he or she must be free to respond or not, each of us is at the same time charged to be responsible for our responses and responsive to the person's concerns—which, I suggest, is the core sense of respect in its moral form.

Perhaps, at least in contemporary times, we can say no more than this: by being open and available (in Marcel's term, *disponible*) to the other by insistently calling for the other's recognition and participation in the patient's search for sense, clinical dialogue itself is enabled and thereby are we willy-nilly collaborators in one another's freedom.[22] The fundamental risk at the heart of dialogue is also clear: the person's appeal to understand and be understood may go unheeded, the need for help unattended, violence not averted—Sartre once reminded us in a memorable reference to Faulkner's great novel, *Light in August,* even when the other is brought down to his knees and his captors try to make him less than human, Joe Christmas, as he calls himself, at the last moment, his life seeping from a fatal gash and empty of everything "save consciousness," looks up at his killers with "unfathomable and unbearable eyes."[23]

Such clinical conversations as I have in mind may not occur, or may fail even if tried, whether the stakes are high or not. The other side of availability is vulnerability, at the heart of which are the ever-present temptations of the callous and the malicious. Nevertheless, without Gyges, there could be no Aesculepius—who in turn is constantly confronted with, but ought never yield to, the Gygean temptation.

The dialectic between vulnerability and power harbors an immense hope and a profound risk: hope that some form of help—whether cure or only comfort—will be ready to hand. Risk, too, in that vulnerability may serve only as a wedge into being deceived or coerced. Both hope and risk are united in an urgent need to know along with the other, and in an act of self-disclosure, at the very moment when the self is deeply and unavoidably susceptible and vulnerable: the patient is, as the ancient healers insisted, "all in your hands."

Yet Mr. Oland does not know what is vital for him to know: what, really, does his wife want? Were she able, what would she say, what would she decide? And if he knows all along, as I think he did, do we dare risk making him confront his own resistance and guilt? The very fact of illness or distress compromises both spiritual and bodily abilities, including language, plain talking, and listening. The vulnerability presented by sickness or distress—whether the patient's or those who are close to the patient—makes a clear difference for the kind of talk that goes on. What is this difference?

Talking and Listening, Listening and Talking

During my final conversation with Mr. Oland, he realized that at one point he had been very disturbed at Dr. Langston's words. Not only was he deeply affected by his wife's condition and impending death, but he displayed precisely the sort of vulnerability I have in mind. His distress— evident in every gesture and word—was an appeal for help, sourced in his love and concern for her and his feeling that Dr. Langston wanted to "force things," as he put it.

He said, "He told me that since she didn't have a living will, and I couldn't tell him anything about what she wanted done, there . . . well, he said he just couldn't or might not be able to do anything for her. Of course, you know, Myra and I had talked some and she did try to get me involved in some of these matters, to get into those things, but even though it was so hard for me to take it or even to listen to her, I still *knew* what she wanted. It's just that, well, you know, that doctor seemed so impatient with me . . . and all I could think about was how I didn't want Myra to talk about those things, didn't want either of us to think about it. So all I could do is sort of blurt out that I didn't know. And then get all mad, 'cause I knew, though . . . oh, yeah, I knew, and we really agreed; I know, too, she knew that's exactly how I felt, too, but I never wanted her to have to face the thing, and didn't really know that I couldn't take it myself. But there are lots of feelings that are so hard to put into words, especially if you've never had the feeling before, and I just couldn't bring myself to really say what I knew."

"I think I understand, Mr. Oland," I tried to respond to the challenge in his words. "Still, I hope you realize that Dr. Langston really should know about this; he's been very disturbed, too, thinking, I suspect, that he somehow managed to offend you—something he'd never want to do. If you want, I'll talk with him, but at some point you really need to talk with him."

"Why? I mean, things are resolved now, aren't they?"

"Obviously, in a sense. But even so, I think it is important for you to tell him what you've told me. He needs to hear it from you; this could help him, and it could also help you too."

"That's not going to be easy, 'cause things got kinda hot and sticky there for a bit, you know? I mean, like I told Janice, that doctor, I thought, was just trying to force things on us, on me. It's kinda like he was, well, you could say, trying to get me to tell him it's okay to let her go, and I just couldn't do that, not then, not ever if I had to do the whatever. I just couldn't live with myself. So, like I said, things got a bit hot, and I even accused him of trying to get me to kill Myra."

"I heard. But, you know, Dr. Langston also felt really bad, even awkward, and he has had difficulty getting things settled in his own mind too. From what I know he thinks that . . . but, really, I shouldn't talk for him; he needs to speak for himself. I can be a go-between only so much."

"I suppose you're right, so I guess I'd best find and talk with him."

Our conversation tapered off then, and I left, knowing that I, too, had to talk with Dr. Langston myself.

As he told me when I finally got to see him, "He just kept insisting that we 'do everything possible.'" He took this to mean that Mr. Oland was "confused" and "inappropriate"; he was really worried that he might be involved in another of those awful cases in which family members push for "doing everything" when, in actuality, "everything" in any reasonable sense has already been done. Later, he was amazed that Mr. Oland had thought that he, Dr. Langston, was trying to "force" things.[24] In any case, they did talk for some time, and both felt that things had been straightened out.

Imperatives of Plain Talk

Kurt Wolff once pointed out that certain imperatives of plain talk are integral to the need to know and do, especially in times of crisis. Indeed, talking about the issue may signify that the person is no longer trapped by it.[25] As I see it, when one gives voice to matters that are crucial and urgent, as in times of serious illness, one turns immediately to others. In such times, the vital need is at once to *understand* and to *be understood*, to know and be known, so that one can try to surmount the experiential urgency that invariably accompanies the illness. In Ortega y Gasset's words, one needs to know what to reckon with (What's wrong? How long will I hurt? What can be done about it?), which in itself sets out a course of seeking: you do *whatever* must be done in order to find out whatever it may be.

In short, facing the crisis of serious illness can bring about a kind of *discipline* whose source is the need to surmount, to resolve, or otherwise overcome the critical matter so that life, as we say, can go on. But seeking, of course, doesn't guarantee finding.[26] Still, if and when you do actually come across what it is imperative to know and understand, that happening occurs most often as a *gift*.

Sometimes, though not always, the gift of understanding, of insight, happens; and when it does, the experience of seeking and finding brings with it a mood of wonder and humility, of relief and gratitude, when we eventually come through or recover from some illness or injury.[27] And this happening, I suggest, includes appeals to other people. To tell others is to invite them to listen, and to ask them also to talk.

This critical need to know is invariably passionate in its utterance. The language of vital need is thus the *passion* that seeks another's *com-passion*; the appeal is for the other to be both responsive and responsible. The passion of the one is coupled with the compassion of the other in the bonds of responsibility. The plight of being a patient in itself solicits (even while it may not receive) compassion, seeking understanding evokes the need for being understanding and being understood (which may not occur), suffering elicits sufferance (again, which may not happen). The Olands' impasse elicited compassionate response. Compassion is, I think, the fundamental form of *availability* to the other,[28] and solicits *trust*—but there, too, is Gyges, whose voice is a temptation to violate the other and yet serves as the clear reminder of the moral worth of the other, whose vulnerability puts us under the governance of its imperatives.

NOTES

I have studied these and related matters for some years. A very early version of this reflection appeared as "Encountering the Other" in: *Duties to Others*, ed. Courtney S. Campbell and B. Andrew Lustig, Theology and Medicine Series (Boston: Kluwer Academic Publishers, 1994), 17–38. Two of my published articles are related to the issues addressed in the present version: "Integrity and Vulnerability in Clinical Medicine: The Dialectic of Appeal and Response," in *Bioethics and Biolaw*, vol. 2, *Four Ethical Principles*, ed. Peter Kemp, Jacob Rendtorff, and Niels Mattsson Johnsen (Copenhagen, Den.: Rhodos International Science and Art Publishers and Centre for Ethics and Law, 2000), 123–40; and "Power and Hope in the Clinical Encounter: A Meditation on Vulnerability," *Medicine, Health Care and Philosophy* 3 (2000): 265–75. This brief narrative is taken from an earlier version that appeared in my book *Troubled Voices: Stories of Ethics and Illness* (Cleveland, OH: Pilgrim Press, 1993); an expanded version of it appeared in my book *Conversations on the Edge: Narratives of Ethics and Illness* (Washington, DC: Georgetown University Press, 2004).

1. Jan van den Berg, *Medical Power and Medical Ethics* (New York: W. W. Norton, 1978).

2. Edmund Husserl, *Cartesian Meditations* (1950; repr., The Hague: Martinus Nijhoff, 1960), §3.

3. A fundamental form of what he terms *"Du-Einstellung."* See Alfred Schutz, *Collected Papers*, vol. 2, *Studies in Social Theory*, Phaenomenologica 15 (The Hague: Martinus Nijhoff, 1964), 161, 173; Alfred Schutz and Thomas Luckmann, *The Structures of the Life-World* (Evanston, IL: Northwestern University Press, 1973), 67–98.

4. See Herbert Plügge, "Man and His Body," in *The Philosophy of the Body*, ed. S. F. Spicker (Chicago: Quadrangle Books, 1970), 296 (originally published as H. Plügge *Der Mensch und sein Leib* [Tübingen: Max Niemeyer Verg, 1967]).

5. Schutz and Luckmann, *The Structures of the Life-World*.

6. Richard M. Zaner, *The Context of Self* (Athens: Ohio University Press, 1981), 227–41.

7. For a more detailed explication of this, see my *Ethics and the Clinical Encounter* (Lima, OH: Academic Renewal Press, 2003), chap. 2 (originally published by Prentice Hall, 1986).

8. See the interesting analysis by Arthur Kleinman, *The Illness Narratives: Suffering, Healing and the Human Condition* (New York: Basic Books, 1988).

9. See Richard M. Zaner, "The Phenomenon of Trust in the Patient-Physician Relationship," in *Ethics, Trust, and the Professions: Philosophical and Cultural Aspects*, ed. E. D. Pellegrino (Washington, DC: Georgetown University Press, 1991), 45–67.

10. Ludwig Edelstein, *Ancient Medicine* (Baltimore: Johns Hopkins University Press, 1967), 329. My reading of the Hippocratic tradition is deeply indebted to the seminal work of this great medical historian.

11. Ibid., 6–30.

12. R. M. Zaner, "Thinking about Medicine," in *Handbook of Phenomenology and Medicine*, ed. S. Kay Toombs (Dordrecht, Neth.: Kluwer Academic Publishers, 2001), 127–44.

13. Plato, *The Republic*, in *The Collected Dialogues*, ed. E. Hamilton and H. Cairns, Book 2, Bollingen Series 71 (Princeton, NJ: Princeton University Press, 1961), 605–30.

14. Hans Jonas, "Toward an Ontological Grounding of an Ethics for the Future," in *Mortality and Morality: A Search for the Good after Auschwitz*, ed. Lawrence Vogel (Evanston, IL: Northwestern University Press, 1996), 101–3.

15. To which there may or may not be a caring response, or any response whatever. What is solicited may not be returned. See Herbert Spiegelberg, "Ethics for Fellows in the Fate of Existence," in *Steppingstones toward an Ethics for Fellow Existers: Essays, 1944–1983* (Dordrecht, Neth.: Martinus Nijhoff, 1986), 199–218, and my *Ethics and the Clinical Encounter*, chap. 11.

16. A term I use to suggest the complex sense of response (responsiveness to and responsibility for) set in caution and vigilance, but with a sense of needing to act.

17. Hans Jonas, *The Imperative of Responsibility: In Search of an Ethics for the Technological Age* (Chicago: University of Chicago Press, 1984), 25–50, 79–109.

158   RICHARD M. ZANER

18. Herbert Spiegelberg, "Good Fortune Obligates: Albert Schweitzer's Second Ethical Principle," *Ethics* 85 (1975): 232.

19. Which is, I think, precisely the powerful point of Gabriel Marcel's rich concept of *disponibilité*. See my "The Mystery of the Body-Qua-Mine," in *The Philosophy of Gabriel Marcel*, ed. P. Schilpp and L. Hahn, Living Library of Philosophy (Carbondale, IL: Open Court Publishing /Southern Illinois University Press, 1984), 313–33.

20. Schutz and Luckmann, *Structures of the Life-World*, 86–225.

21. Alfred Schutz, "The Stranger: An Essay in Social Psychology," in *Collected Papers II: Studies in Social Theory* (The Hague: Martinus Nijhoff, 1964).

22. Gabriel Marcel, *Metaphysical Journal* (Chicago: Henry Regnery, 1952), 30–31, 234–35; also, Gabriel Marcel, *Du Refus á l'invocation* (Paris: Gallimard, 1940).

23. William Faulkner, *Light in August* (1932; repr., New York: Modern Library, 1959), 470.

24. This is an interesting example of the kind of violation mentioned earlier: clearly, although ultimately recognized as a "misunderstanding," Mr. Oland experienced and reacted to Dr. Langston's talk as coercive.

25. K. Wolff, *Surrender and Catch: Experience and Inquiry Today* (Boston: D. Reidel Publishing, 1976), 31.

26. Zaner, *Context of Self*, 181–98.

27. Zaner, *Ethics and the Clinical Encounter*, chap. 2.

28. As Gabriel Marcel urged many times, this availability (*disponibilité*: being of avail, at the disposal of, the other person) is the key notion to authentic interpersonal relationships; see *Du refus à l'invocation*, esp. 55–80, 192–225.

CHAPTER

9

Vulnerability within the Body of Christ
Anointing of the Sick and Theological Anthropology

M. Therese Lysaught

The philosophical anthropology that dominates medicine and bioethics too often reduces human identity to rationality and autonomy individualistically construed. Yet for such an anthropology, the realities of illness—a sine qua non of medicine and bioethics—stand as anomalies. Illness quickly marshals empirical evidence against its truth claims.

Rather than standing as a confounding glitch, illness and healing have been central to the Christian tradition since its beginning. What one finds in early Christian sources is easy to miss or dismiss, given our habit of reading such narratives and practices with lenses shaped by modern philosophy. But if we listen carefully to these sources, we will, I submit, discover a more accurate and adequate account of who we are and what it means for us to flourish. This chapter stands as a first step in developing a more truthful anthropology for bioethics, namely, a *theological* anthropology.

Healing and the Kingdom of God

A theological anthropology for bioethics cannot but begin with the Gospels. To state the obvious, in the Gospels, Jesus heals the sick.[1] Until the Passion, healing is one of his signature actions, along with preaching, teaching, and the occasional multiplication of loaves. But the less obvious question is this: Why do the gospel writers focus so much attention on Jesus' healing activities? Why, in sending out his disciples, did Jesus command them to heal the sick? Why does healing loom so large in Jesus' project?

Three passages from Luke help to clarify and complicate this question. Part of the larger narrative of Jesus' life and of God's way of dwelling with the world that begins with the opening chapter of Genesis and extends through the end of Revelation, they are but three of dozens of examples that could be mustered to demonstrate the centrality of healing to that narrative. God, the tradition attests, wills life, wellness, wholeness, and embodied flourishing. Healing is central to the God disclosed in scripture. God's healing, however, is not a generic, disembodied concept. "Healing" cannot simply be affirmed, lifted out of scripture, and filled with just any content. The scriptural narrative gives God's relationship to healing a very particular, very complex shape.

Consider Luke 7, where Jesus responds to John the Baptist's query whether Jesus is "he who is to come, or shall we look for another?" Is Jesus, in other words, the Messiah who will inaugurate the kingdom of God? Jesus replies, "Go and tell John what you have seen and heard: the blind receive their sight, the lame walk, lepers are cleansed, and the deaf hear, the dead are raised up, the poor have good news preached to them. And blessed is he who takes no offense at me" (Luke 7:22–23).[2] Here we hear the familiar tropes—the poor and the sick, healing and raising up, preaching the good news and (obliquely) the kingdom of God. But it ends on a jarring note: clearly, some have taken offense.

Three chapters later, Jesus sends forth seventy-two disciples, two by two, who are to precede him in the places he intends to visit. In doing so, he says to them "Be on your way, and remember: I am sending you as lambs in the midst of wolves. Do not carry a walking staff or a traveling bag; wear no sandals and greet no one along the way. On entering any house, first say 'Peace to this house.' . . . Into whatever city you go, after they welcome you, eat what they set before you, and cure the sick there. Say to them, 'The reign of God is at hand'" (Luke 10:1–9). Again the healing of the sick is connected to the *evangel*, the good news of the in-breaking of the kingdom of God. But again, conflict lurks: he sends them as lambs in the midst of wolves. Their first word, the word to frame their practice of healing and preaching of the kingdom, is *peace*.

These interconnections burst forth boldly in chapter 11, the heart of Luke's narrative:

> Jesus was driving out a demon that was mute, and when the demon had gone out, the mute man spoke and the crowds were amazed. Some of them said, "By the power of Beelzebul, the prince of demons, he drives out demons." Others, to test him, asked him for a sign from heaven. But he knew their thoughts and said to them, "Every kingdom divided against itself will be laid waste and house will fall against house. And if Satan is divided against himself, how will his kingdom stand? For you say that it is by Beelzebul that I drive out demons. If I, then, drive out demons by Beelzebul, by whom do your own people drive them out? Therefore they will be your judges. But if it is by the finger of God that I drive out demons, then the Kingdom of God has come upon you. When a strong man fully armed guards his palace, his possessions are safe. But when one stronger than he attacks and overcomes him, he takes away the armor on which he relied and distributes the spoils. Whoever is not with me is against me, and whoever does not gather with me scatters." (Luke 11:14–23)

What has been hinted at up to this point now becomes clear—that within the Gospels, practices of healing are overlaid with political valence.[3] In John's gospel, Jesus' acts of healing are one of the reasons the religious authorities seek to kill him. Yet here, in Luke's gospel, because of his healing actions, the authorities accuse Jesus of consorting with the enemy! Jesus, in response, claims that his healing practices presuppose, presage, reveal, and are coincident with a particular social order—nothing less than the kingdom of God. One author goes so far as to note that "the two ideas [healing and the kingdom] are so constantly coupled, by Jesus or the gospel writers, that one might almost call [the mission of healing] their definition of the Kingdom of God."[4]

Healing, in short, is deeply intertwined with the presence, proclamation, and politics of the kingdom of God. And readers are called to make a choice. With which kingdom are they going to side? "Whoever is not with me is against me, and whoever does not gather with me scatters." In making that choice, in siding with God's kingdom, those who are "with" Jesus find practices of healing to be central to the ways of discipleship. Healing is a central part of the commission Jesus gives to those he sends out into the world to preach the good news of the kingdom and to embody it wherever they go. But this is not simply healing qua healing.[5] Healing, which is of the kingdom, prepares the way for Jesus' coming and is always linked to the proclamation and embodiment of the kingdom; it is inextricably linked to peace (yet another political concept). The Gospels, then, portray healing as politically charged, inextricably connected to the kingdom of God.

Illness, Vulnerability and Politics: A Brief Phenomenology

But if healing is thus connected, what about illness? Acts of healing presume a substrate of sick human bodies. It is upon the bodies of the sick that this political drama—the drama of the stronger man attacking and overcoming the one who is well-armed—is being played out. As their bodies are healed, others feel threatened and take offense. Bodies, in other words, are the site at which power is being contested. Is being ill in and of itself somehow "political"? How might healing and the polis, bodies and the social order, be connected?

To address this question, briefly consider the notion of "vulnerability."[6] To be vulnerable, in the strict sense of the word, is to be susceptible to being wounded, to be open to attack or damage (from the Latin, f. *vulner-*, *vulnus* wound). In some ways, *vulnerable* is an odd word to apply to the sick— clearly, their "defenses" have already been breached;[7] they have already been wounded. Yet illness not only makes clear that vulnerability is an ineradicable dimension of human existence but also makes clear that to sustain one wound is to become open to further wounding—in fact, to become open to an almost snowball effect of injury on almost every other level.

Wounds are given. They come from outside of us. To be wounded requires an agent or an agency. In illness, although the initial "wound" comes quite often from an impersonal source (e.g., a pathogen), subsequent "wounds" often come at the hands of others. With the advent of illness, we become subject to the power of others in a radical way. Likewise, the ameliorating of woundedness or protection therefrom also necessarily comes at the hands of others. The sick find themselves suspended in a complex web of social interactions, a web of practices configuring and configured by a social order.

This briefest reflection on vulnerability, then, almost immediately suggests connections to a "politics." Such a connection is confirmed when one turns to accounts offered by those who have experienced illness or cared for sick and suffering persons. These narratives quickly display how the "wound" of illness spirals the sick through successive levels of vulnerability, leading to further experiences of loss or woundedness exacerbated by the mostly covert exercise of power. The first draft of this chapter drew on illness narratives to provide thick descriptions of four successive "wounds" of illness: marginalization and isolation, hyper-identification with yet simultaneous alienation from the body, usurpation of "voice," and discounted rationality. However, Kay Toombs's chapter earlier in this volume wonderfully displays these dynamics.[8] Thus I gladly defer to her phenomenology and will focus here on the interrelationships between bodies and polities.

Toombs's phenomenology incisively illustrates how isolating and marginalizing illness can be. The "wound" of illness renders vulnerable both our "place" and our "visibility." Not only does such marginalization result from biological factors; equally, the social isolation that attends illness can reflect social intolerance or fear of weakness and imperfection. Others' illnesses remind us of our own vulnerability, our own contingency. Those who understand themselves fundamentally as autonomous beings do not want to be so reminded of the contingency of their control.

Nor does society want to be reminded of this contingency. Culture, basing its self-esteem on the ability to keep nature at bay, fears the "chaotic" powers of nature that, though repressed, threaten to explode from their bonds; only nature in aesthetically pleasing and culturally ordered forms is given public space. Thus, as Toombs notes, physical and temporal structures of public social life reflect this resistance, effectively discouraging participation from those who become ill.

The "wound" of illness, then, renders us vulnerable to further wounding on the social level. At a time when our need for companionship is greatest because of increased dependence, we often find ourselves relocated out of the public purview, avoided by others, internalizing others' fear of our wounded bodies.

Toombs describes well how pain or illness often makes us conscious of our bodies in new ways, experiencing it as more present yet also profoundly alien. Toombs likewise notes how, in the face of this biologically mediated wounding of the relationship between body and self, the human agency embodied in medical care often exacerbates the injury. When the sick bring this tension and destabilizing reversal of body/self roles to medical encounters, medical practitioners, rather than countering this alienation, often reify a dualistic reading of body-self interrelationship. Not only are most modern medical encounters structured so that there is little time for physicians to do other than attend to the presented physical ailment, medical practitioners are habituated to identify patients primarily or only with their bodies or diseases (the "dysfunction" of their body); medicine often reduces patients to specific diagnoses of disease.

Derivative of these levels of vulnerability, the sick can also find their "voice" threatened in expected and unexpected ways. Voice may literally be lost as a function of pain or infirmity, or legitimate "voice" may be denied or repressed because it does not fit with normative medical or moral language. Yet again, medicine, rather than counteracting this vulnerability of voice following from the initial "wound" of illness, often exacerbates it. As many have noted, vis-à-vis medicine, patients find themselves "strangers in a strange land."[9] In order to participate in the healing process, patients must conform themselves to the customs of medicine and learn its languages, rather than vice versa; patients' lack of knowledge of the "language" of medicine can intimidate them, leaving them "speechless." Further, medicine not only effectively suppresses the voice of the sick, but at times often actively usurps it. All too often, patients' interpretations of the symptoms of their illness are taken away from them by medicine and translated into the language of the profession: "For the practitioner, the patient's complaints (symptoms of illness) must be translated into the *signs* of disease."[10] Physicians often feel that they have to read between the lines, to distill meaning from confused and messy narratives of patients, to make "subjective" experiences of patients' illnesses into "objective" categorized diseases. Patients, along with their voices, are rendered inadequate, unhelpful, wrong, and silenced.

The final assault that the "wound" of illness can bring threatens what has come to be considered the very core of our human identity, the sine qua non that establishes us as "persons" and protects us under the penumbra of civilly guaranteed rights. Succinctly put, the sick are often perceived as being rationally "impaired" or "deficient" because of the emotive and physical dimensions of their condition.

As noted, medical practitioners have been taught to regard with *suspicion* patients' illness narratives. They sift out meaning from patients' accounts, listening selectively "so that some aspects are carefully listened for and heard (sometimes when they are not spoken), while other things that are said—and even repeated—are literally not heard."[11] At times, patients' claims of illness or pain are doubted, if not explicitly denied, especially in the cases of chronically ill patients or in cases where the "explanatory framework" of medicine has not yet shifted to allow an illness into "reality."[12] Alternatively, patients who reject a diagnosis of disease, or who do not conform to acceptable modes of dealing with a diagnosis, may be labeled as "in denial"; physiological interpretations are given higher epistemic status than patient's lived experiential interpretations. Thus the ontological assault of illness is interpreted as disabling rationality. As H. Tristram Engelhardt notes, "Patients often regress under the stress of disease and come to be treated and want to be treated as children."[13]

In illness then, the initial "wound" of illness ripples out to unveil a network of interconnected vulnerabilities, compounding injury with injury: the sick become isolated and marginalized, become alienated from their very bodies, lose their "voice," and find their minds discounted. The cumulative impact of these injuries is simple: in illness, we can find our very selves dissolved. As Reynolds Price, rendered paraplegic in midlife, notes, "your main want . . . is simply *the person you used to be*. But you're not that person now. . . . [Your old self] is dead as any teen-aged Marine drilled through the forehead in an Asian jungle; any Navy Seal with his legs blown off, halved for the rest of the time he gets. . . . Reynolds Price is dead."[14]

Yet such dissolution cannot be reduced to biology, nor can it be construed as primarily an individual, existential event. For, as the foregoing phenomenology indicates, such dissolution of the self is politically mediated. Each successive wounding occurs through the agency of others or the very structures of our social order. To be sick is to be "politically incorrect" in a most profound way. To be sick is to literally embody—make clear in visibly heightened ways—a radically different account of reality. Sick bodies are "unruly" (to use language current in disabilities studies). They do not conform to normative social meanings. They challenge those readings of the world that our culture puts forward as "truths."[15] Weakness, dependence, and imperfection are not part of the story our culture tells us about itself; these realities are deeply at odds with contemporary values of efficiency, productivity, physical beauty, and perfection. The reality of suffering and the inability of the sick to control their bodies are equally despised and feared. We who have been so deeply formed by the myth that we are autonomous beings do not want to be reminded of the radical contingency of our control over nature, over our lives, over our destinies. The radical lack of autonomy or the undeniable realities of dependence of the sick challenge a society grounded in the "truths" of autonomy and self-sufficiency.

Illness reminds us that we are in fact embodied, hardly the Cartesian selves, the disincarnate minds that we prefer to think we are. And few dynamics of illness could be more dangerous in our culture than loss of voice—so central to our sense of agency—or loss of rationality or autonomy, without which we effectively become nonpersons. In short, the sick (literally) embody the antithesis of our culture.

The sick, then, find themselves in the most radically vulnerable position. The vulnerability of their bodies opens a point of vulnerability for the social order. Through their "wound," the social body likewise finds itself threatened with multiple and successive levels of wounding. The whole house of cards might collapse. Such challenges must be decisively met. Bodies that manifest such alternate truths or realities must be reinscribed with dominant social truths or relocated in such a way that their challenge is minimized or eliminated. To meet this "dis-inscription" of deeply embodied social truths requires equally deeply embodied practices.

Since Foucault, medicine has been understood as a major agent of this process. Through the array of practices it performs on bodies, medicine functions to reinscribe them with the meanings of the social order—to reinscribe, in other words, a particular anthropology.[16] Medicine often succeeds in reconstructing sick bodies to fit with social norms. But not always. Individuals that medicine cannot make fit into the "truths" of the social order find themselves pushed to the margins of society or beyond. Those whose suffering can be controlled but not defeated—the disabled, the chronically ill—people the margins. Those whose suffering cannot be controlled, whose bodies cannot be reinscribed, are increasingly encouraged or assisted—through practices such as physician-assisted suicide—to exit beyond the boundaries, all under the rubric of dominant social values such as autonomy, self-sufficiency, and control. Unruly bodies thus disappear, and the social order is purged of the threat.

Anointing the Sick: An Alternative Politics

Healing practices, then, are political. They function in part to validate—embody, make real—particular social norms, thereby continuing to instantiate a particular polis, and they function to take hold of human bodies and locate them within the proper place in the social sphere. Alternative practices might therefore be perceived as profoundly socially destabilizing, politically threatening. They might give offense. They might provoke violence (or at least get people taken to court).

In the Gospels, as we have seen, Jesus' practice of healing is explicitly linked to an alternative polity, the kingdom of God. The early church recognized that the bodies of the sick presented a key locus for practicing and embodying the Christian life and for making the kingdom of God real in the world, both corporeally and corporately. Without the benefit of Foucault, they realized the power of illness to introduce vulnerability into the social order of the ecclesial community. Following Jesus' own healing practice, they intuited that the primary response to this very real threat must be an embodied practice, a practice that (literally) touches bodies in order to reinscribe them within particular truths and social norms. Thus the early church anointed the sick.

The practice of anointing provides an important theological starting point for meditating on anthropology and bioethics. Today the practice remains one of the few spaces where the religious/theological irrupts—visually, tactilely, practically—into the domain of modern medicine, even within secular hospitals. In this way, it provides an almost indispensable starting point for thinking theologically in the realm of medicine and bioethics. At the same time, despite deformations through the centuries, the practice of anointing the sick has endured as a key ecclesial practice. Elevated to the status of a sacrament within the Catholic tradition, the practice of anointing stands as the church's primary response to the event of illness and the unfolding vulnerabilities it presents. Moreover, insofar as practices are important epistemological loci—through them we come to *know* what we believe (in this case, what we believe theologically about the human person), and correlatively, it is only through our practices that we can enact what we profess to believe (i.e., our "ethic")—it is to practices that we ought to look for our anthropological claims.[17]

A complete account of the practice of anointing would attend to its historical development, its contemporary enactments, and so forth, which unfortunately is beyond the parameters of this chapter. For our purposes, I will explore one early account of anointing, the traditional warrant for the practice found in James 5:14–16: "Is anyone among you ill? Let that person call the elders of the assembly, and let them, after anointing him with oil in the name of the Lord, pray over the person. And the prayer of faith will save the sick person, and the Lord will raise him up. And if the person has committed sins, he will be forgiven. Therefore, confess sins to each other and pray for each other so that you may be healed."[18] How might this passage lead us to key theological insights crucial for shaping an anthropology for medicine and bioethics? How might the way Christians care for the sick illuminate what we affirm to be central about human identity?

James's Rhetorical Structure

Recent New Testament scholarship has rehabilitated the Letter of James against centuries of rejection and marginalization. Long cast as one of the latest New Testament writings, more recent readings suggest that the letter is in fact one of the earliest. Recent scholarship has also dashed the long-traditional reading that the letter is simply a loose compilation of disconnected aphorisms and moral exhortations. Most critics now argue that James possesses not only internal coherence and argument but a compelling vision of the contours of the Christian life.

Luke Timothy Johnson locates the letter's central rhetorical pivot in verse 4:4 where James charges, "Do you not know that friendship with the world is enmity with God? Therefore, whoever chooses to be a friend of the world is established as an enemy of God." This fundamental polarity between "friendship with the world," which is enmity with God, and "friendship with God" is the central principle that organizes and shapes James's message from start to finish. Throughout the letter, such friendship and allegiance is presented not as an ontologically given—not, for example, a matter of ethnic identity (i.e., because one is Jewish)—but rather as a matter of individual and communal choice.

What would it have meant to be "friends of the world"? "Friendship" in the Greco-Roman context was an extraordinarily rich category, carrying much greater weight than the term carries today. "To have friends," Johnson notes, "meant above all to share: to have the same mind, the same outlook, the same view of reality."[19] Those familiar with Aristotle, for example, will recall that in the *Nichomachean Ethics*, the friendship of equals is the highest form of love, much more crucial for the polis than friendship between unequals or even that least of friendship between the most unequals, romantic or marital love. Friendship was the glue that held the polis together.

To be "friends of the world," then, meant to participate in a particular view of reality, of the way things are, a sharing that was simultaneously cognitive and political. The "world," for James, does not connote nature or creation, or some neutral space of human activity, or what we might call "the public sphere." Johnson describes it, rather, as a logic, a system of valuing or measurement, that plays itself out in actions and practices. He characterizes this as the logic of "envy, rivalry, competition, and murder."[20] As he notes, for James, the measure of the world "is defined precisely in terms of the logic of envy. Human existence is a zero-sum game in a universe of limited resources, a closed system. Being and worth are dependent on having; having more means being more, and having less means being less. By this logic, humans are essentially in competition with each other for being and worth, and the surest way to succeed is to eliminate the competition."[21] To be "friends of the world," then, is to share this worldview, to see reality in these terms. It is to believe that the world is a closed system, a universe of limited resources, and it is to live as if this were true—to live in competition, in rivalry, in maximizing one's share of scarce resources, even if my accumulation means that others go without, even if it means, because of this, their death.

To be "friends of God," in contrast, means something altogether different. To be "friends of God" is to share God's mindset, God's view of reality, God's "wisdom" (in the language of the letter), and God's corresponding way of being and acting in the world. As is stated almost at the beginning of the letter (in James 1:5, and repeated in 1:17 and 4:6), the essential attribute of God is gift, is giving: "God," James proclaims, "continually gives. . . . God does not restrict giving only to those who make requests, but simply gives 'to all.'"[22]

To be a friend of God, then, is to know and celebrate the fundamental character of reality, to proclaim this marvelous truth—that God exists, that God is true, and that, consequently, the fundamental context of existence is gift—open, abundant, for-the-other rather than against-the-other. As Johnson notes, "James['s] real distinctiveness comes in the breathtaking assertion—grounded in the symbolic world of Torah shared by every form of Judaism including the nascent movement rooted in the 'faith of Jesus Christ'—that human existence is not located within a closed system of competition (even for virtue or excellence) but rather within an open system ordered to a God who gives gifts to humanity. This is the theological perspective of 'faith.'" Thus, James renarrates reality in a fundamentally theological way. He tells a different story about the way things are, and he challenges his community to inhabit and live within that story, which is the story of God.

Friendship with God and friendship with the world are thus mutually exclusive perspectives. To be a friend of God is to reject the world's way of construing reality and to reject the violence that it necessarily entails. It is to be a person whose essential nature, whose entire character, is oriented toward giving, not only to those who ask but simply "to all." Those who choose to side with "the world," however, are not simply and relativistically inhabiting a different story—they are choosing to be "*enemies* of God."

For to see reality differently means to live in reality differently. Indeed, James reserves his most scathing invective not so much for those who are "friends with the world," but for those who are "double-minded"—those who want to have it both ways.[23]

Money, Community, Suffering, and Prayer

This rhetorical framework sets the context for rereading James's more familiar elements. Four in particular are important as we move toward the practice of anointing at the end of the letter. First is James's famous acerbic critique of socioeconomic inequities. Signaled from the very opening of the letter,[24] James particularly castigates those who practice economic favoritism *within* the assembly, for what could be worse than finding enmity with God practiced within and by the very community that names itself friend of God?[25] The vast disparities between the rich and the poor, and particularly enculturated behaviors toward both, is the primary area in which we see what it means in practice to live as "friends with the world" rather than as "friends with God." For if God is preeminently the one who gives to all unstintingly, then to amass wealth is to display disbelief in God; to amass wealth when others have little or nothing is to position oneself as God's enemy. Indeed, toward the end of the letter he produces his greatest invective for the rich, raining down woes on their heads for defrauding laborers of their wages.[26] For acquiring such wealth can only occur within the logic of the world, which requires injustice, and the essence of this injustice is violence and, indeed, "murder."

The lives of those who call themselves friends of God will be characterized by economic sharing.[27] For the view of reality that God gives all to all does not exist apart from embodied actions that make the claim true. Thus, in the community that styles itself as a friend of God, radical socioeconomic inequities are no more. The lowly are "raised up," the rich are "humbled." To say that one believes in God but does not live this belief—does not materially care for the needs of one's brothers and sisters—is to prove one's claims to faith to be empty.

The framework of friendship with God versus friendship with the world likewise undergirds a second subtheme, namely, the *ekklesia* as a "community of solidarity." James is often misread, saying that his injunctions are directed toward individuals and that the point of his exhortations is to move individuals toward moral perfection. The author of James, however, is thoroughgoingly communitarian. From verse 1, James uses plural pronouns and addresses his audience as an *"ekklesia."*[28] James, in other words, exhorts the *community* to embody a particular identity; he exhorts the *community* to inhabit and "realize" the truth of the story of God.

Friendship with the world requires us to see ourselves as individuals. The logic of the world, the logic of competition, presumes two diametrically opposed players, locked in a zero-sum game of win-lose. The "other" is a threat to me, a threat of loss, a threat of subjection and oppression, a threat to my very life. To survive requires that I "look out for number one." But a world grounded in a God who gives all to all requires a different anthropology. Fundamental to a theo-logic of giving is a radically inverted and egalitarian mutuality. For all stand before God, equal in need, equal in giftedness. There is no competition for God's grace and providence. James calls his hearers to see themselves not as individuals in competition but as brothers and sisters in Christ, equal members of a community of solidarity created and sustained by God's grace. Certainly James calls each member of the community "to behavior consonant with the community's" professed identity, but he is most interested in creating "a community of solidarity," one that makes "the choice between a life of envy that logically tends toward the elimination of the other in murder and a life based on gift and mercy expressed in service of the other."[29]

This communitarian nature of friendship with God undergirds the third subtheme, namely, James's oft-misinterpreted references to endurance of suffering and testings. Indeed, the letter opens with this very theme in 1:2–4: "My brothers and sisters, consider it entirely joy whenever you encounter various testings, since you know that the testing of your *faith* produces endurance. And let endurance yield a perfect product, in order that you might be perfect and complete, lacking in nothing" (emphasis mine). Too often this passage is read, like much of the rest of James, as exhorting individual endurance in the face of suffering. Yet again we return to James's context and framework. The testing of the *community's* faith (for again, here, the pronoun is plural) would be the testing of its theological read of reality, its proclamation that God is God and that God gives all to all. Testings, then, are challenges to the community's attempt to live the story of God, to faithfully embody their conviction that God is the truth of reality.

James returns to the theme of suffering as the letter draws to a close. At the outset he counseled "joy." Here, in the face of testings, he counsels them four times in four lines (5:7–11) to "be patient." They will be oppressed;

they will be scorned; the world will try to introduce dissension into the community. Patience in the face of these testings will produce endurance, which brings blessing. But even more, patience is not simply quiet endurance of suffering. It is the embodiment of God's patient and nonviolent way with the world as well as the affirmation of God's ultimate providence.

Last we come to James's remarks that run throughout the letter on the proper and improper uses of speech. Not only does he caution his comrades against becoming teachers and rail against the poisonous nature of the tongue (3:1–12), but throughout he identifies both negative and positive functions of speech. The proscribed modes of speech are many.[30] These evidence "friendship with the world," the speaker's attempt to assert the self at the expense of others and of the truth.

The final section of the letter (5:12–20), on the other hand, exhorts the community to a variety of positive modes of speech. "How can the tongue be used not for the destruction of humans," Johnson asks, "but for the building up of a community of solidarity?" These simple uses of speech—plain talk, prayer, confessing, correcting—demonstrate that speech can be not only an instrument of envy, competition, and violence but also one of peace, cooperation, and solidarity.

Such speech is possible, of course, only in light of God's speech or "word." God's relational, indeed, covenantal "word of truth" (1:18) has brought into being this distinctive community, this "first fruits," this community whose identity and behavior differ markedly from the "wisdom" of the world.[31] And it is prayer—that mode of speech that preeminently affirms James's theological construal of reality—that is essential for helping the community and its members to perceive God's truth. *Lex orandi, lex credendi.* As we pray, so we believe. By enacting a belief, we come to understand it and to truly believe it. Consequently, as Johnson notes, "It is surely not by accident that James' composition begins and ends on the topic of prayer, since prayer is the activity that most fundamentally defines and expresses that construal of reality called 'faith.'"[32] It is only by speaking rightly, in other words, that we learn to see.

Rereading Anointing

These five aspects of the Letter of James, then—his overarching exhortation to friendship with God rather than with the world, lived as a community of solidarity shaped by radical socioeconomic egalitarianism, that consequently bears the enmity of the world peaceably with joy and patience as a way of embodying both confidence in God and God's way in the world and performs faith and solidarity through act and word—provide the context by which to reread the practice of anointing the sick.

The passage that contains reference to anointing (James 5:12–20) is, as mentioned earlier, James's closing exhortation on prayer and positive modes of speech within the community. Anointing, then, is at the same time a physical action practiced upon sick bodies, which is simultaneously a mode of speech. Speech for James, of course, is not simply verbal but performative, expressed in action (see 1:22–25; 2:14–26).

This nexus of touch/speech/prayer singled out in the context of illness returns us to our earlier analysis of illness, vulnerability, and politics. For as much as anointing is a practice for the sick person, it is equally an action about and for the community. Notably, the context of James's exhortation to prayer is specific: the context of sufferings, sickness. Suffering and sickness can powerfully test faith, can powerfully test the truth of the community's theological construal of reality as the story of a present and provident God. As much as illness threatens our modern social order, for very different reasons James likewise understands sickness to pose "a profound threat to the identity and stability of the community."[33]

On the one hand, illness threatens the community with social division and alienation. Scriptural passages testify to the social ramifications that attended illness in Jewish culture—ostracism, associations of uncleanness (alienation from their own bodies) and of punishment from God. But this is simply to follow the logic of the world, whose natural reflex for survival is to isolate the sick from the healthy, to give them a lower social status out of fear of loss. Health, here, is a zero-sum game.

With illness, the community finds itself faced with a situation akin to that of economic inequities. The language surrounding the practice of anointing—that the Lord will "raise the sick person up"—echoes James's opening language of "the lowly brother [being] exalted." While James's use of "raise up" must be heard in its New Testament/Gospel context, where it bears equally physical and eschatological meanings (often both at the same time), for James, "raising up" also clearly connotes the overcoming of social distinctions within the community. The *"ekklesia"* is to anoint the sick precisely to counter the social distinctions and alienation introduced into the community by the advent of illness.

As Johnson notes, sickness challenges the community of faith to make a choice:

Will it behave like friends of God or like friends of the world? According to the wisdom from below, the proper result of fierce competition is survival of the fittest. The logic of envy is to claim strength at the expense of others. Envy, we have seen, leads to murder. Does someone fall sick? They are weak, leave them by the wayside. Their elimination leaves more resources for me; having to share my attention and resources with them distracts me and weakens me for my own struggle for supremacy and survival.[34]

Consequently, James here for the first time uses the term "*ekklesia*," for it is the identity of the community *as* community that sickness threatens. "Will the community rally in support of the weak and show itself to be 'merciful and rich in compassion,' a community based in solidarity, or will it recoil in fear and leave the sick person to progressive alienation?"[35]

More crucially, the practice of anointing is for James an action *of* the "*ekklesia*."[36] With the advent of sickness, the stakes are raised: sickness requires a specifically communal response. Anointing is an action that takes place within the Christian community as the community of faith; it is an action that embodies the communities' claims about its identity as the Body of Christ; it is an action that seeks to reinscribe what it knows as truths on the bodies of the sick. The community faces the test of illness and no longer finds the sick person to be a threat; rather they are reminded that the sick person is a gift, is "entirely joy." In the "wound" of illness—a wound inflicted on both the sick person and the community—the Christian and the "*ekklesia*" find themselves called to continued openness, openness to the continued possibility of wounding rather than embodying the logic of the world, which is to close oneself off, to embody the belief that the world is a closed system. Under the aegis of God, who gives all to all, the sick in their woundedness are no longer seen as alien threats but rather rightly seen as gifts.

Polities and Anthropologies

In anointing the sick, the Christian community faces the threat of vulnerability posed by illness and does not blink. It welcomes into its midst the enemy. Anointing embodies the Christian tradition's refusal to allow suffering, illness, and even death to dissuade it from its faith in God's reality, God's presence, God's goodness, and God's generosity. It embodies the community's refusal to treat the sick according to a logic not of God. Anointing embodies the cross in the confidence of the Resurrection.

Illness tempts the sick and community alike to live not according to the logic of friendship with God but according to the powerfully attractive logic of friendship with the world. For clearly, the logic of friendship with the world can be traced throughout the multiple woundings outlined earlier. Yet anointing stands against this logic. In its collective action as the Body of Christ, the church via anointing the sick counters the cultural effects of isolation and marginalization; anointing witnesses that sick persons are not something to be hidden away.[37] It challenges cultural aversiveness to sick bodies, as well as unattainable cultural norms of bodily perfection, by practicing a witness of touch and blessing. It counters the tendency in the practice of medicine to reduce the patient's voice to a mere matter of consent by both encouraging the patient to summon the church and acting as a surrogate voice of prayer before God (rather than a surrogate voice of choice before the law). And it will counter the construction within medicine of sick persons as, contradictorily, both autonomous individuals and passive recipients of medical ministrations.

By responding to the sick with the practice of anointing, the church affirms that autonomy is not the first and last word; rather, autonomy, control, and their handmaid individualism are hallmarks of what it means to live as friends with the world. With anointing, we discover how deeply we are "members of one another" and how the sick not only are recipients of our care but importantly minister equally to us. They are gifts to the community that enable it to embody God's continued openness in the face of suffering rather than opting for closing, cutting off, and isolating. Those on both sides of the practice of anointing should find themselves liberated from utilitarian frameworks that construe the world as one of limited resources that pit individuals against one another in competition for those scarce resources and that rely on cost-benefit calculations.

No better example of this could be offered than story of the Christian community narrated by Kay Toombs at the end of her chapter. Here we see what it looks like for a Christian community to embody friendship with God vis-à-vis the sick. In doing so, the *"ekklesia"* makes an extraordinary witness to the world. It displays the truth of Christianity, what it means to always see the other as gift—even if the other seems to be a threat to the self or community. It displays trust in God, trust that God is present, and trust that God, who gives all to all, will continue to sustain the sick person as well as the community.

Anointing and the tradition of caring for the sick make possible a decidedly different polity. And it is this polity that enables us to think differently about who we are and what it means to flourish. If nothing else, this analysis calls us to a greater vigilance about the practices of medicine and bioethics. It calls us to question the metaphysical and anthropological claims, the identities and truths they seek to produce in and through the bodies of the sick. It makes clear how deeply subject the sick are to the power of others and how the power exercised through medicine can be deployed either toward the ends of the world—maintaining and fostering the contemporary social order, which too often is one of violence, competition, cost-effectiveness, and profit—or toward the ends of the kingdom of God—a kingdom of nonviolent love, reconciliation, and radical egalitarianism whose ultimate goal is the union of the community as community with God. Especially for those of us in healthcare, it will remind us that real power, the power of God witnessed in the world, is made perfect not through control but through weakness. Will we be with him, he asks, or against him?

NOTES

1. Throughout the chapter I will specify a number of methodological commitments that undergird my argument. Here let me state the first: (1) *The starting point of theological anthropology must be theological.* To start such a venture with an anthropological starting point risks ending up, instead, with anthropological theology, lending credence to Feuerbach's critique. As Catherine LaCugna similarly maintains, "One of the lessons learned from the history of Trinitarian theology is that metaphysical positions must be rooted in and derived from what we know of God as revealed in the economy of salvation. Otherwise, metaphysical claims . . . will appear to be nothing more than projections of human values onto the divine being." Catherine LaCugna, *Freeing Theology* (San Francisco: Harper San Francisco, 1993), 91. In short, the perspective offered here maintains that for a theological anthropology, what we know or affirm about ourselves (anthropology) must be rooted in what we know or affirm about God (theology).

Related to this is a second methodological commitment: (2) *The primary theological starting point for theological anthropology lies in the economy of salvation, that is, the person and work of Jesus Christ.* LaCugna takes to task theological positions that begin philosophically or anthropologically: "In both cases," she notes, "what is usually missing is a firm basis in salvation history—in the person of Jesus Christ—for a particular vision of society" (Ibid., 91), or in our case for particular vision of the human person. Jesus Christ, as the fullness of revelation, stands as the key to interpreting all other modes of revelation and human knowledge, our window into the character of God. The proper starting point of theological anthropology must be Christologically construed.

2. All scriptural citations are from the Revised Standard Version, except the passages from the Letter of James (see note 18).

3. I will use the word *political* in this chapter in the Aristotelian sense, as relating to the polis and the structured social interactions that are both shaped by and required for the maintenance of such a polis. I prefer the word *political* to *social* insofar as the notions of peace and violence associated with gospel healing have more "political" than "social" connotations.

4. Pierson Parker, "Early Christianity as a Religion of Healing," *St. Luke's Journal of Theology* 19 (March 1976): 146.

5. A fuller portrayal of gospel healing accounts would also display, for example, the interconnections between Jesus' acts of healing and the cross, or between Jesus' acts of healing and Israeli-gentile relations, as well as their interconnections to the Jewish scriptures, and so on. Clearly, such a portrayal is beyond the scope of this chapter.

6. An alternative line of analysis to that rooted in vulnerability might be to describe sick persons as "political" agents—even if they are not the "agents" of healing strictly speaking, and even it their agency is not as visibly "active" as the agency of others. Many of the sick in the Gospels do exercise quite a bit of agency— they seek out healing, they ask Jesus for it (or someone close to them does), they persist against his apparent reluctance. I pursue this line of inquiry elsewhere in trying to explore how we might re-envision the practice of anointing as a sacrament of vocation. Importantly, however, to posit the sick as having agency, that agency must—toward the end of theological anthropology—remain carefully connected to the scriptural witness. To take an affirmation of the political centrality/agency of the sick and read it as simply supporting patient autonomy, for example, would be theologically problematic.

7. Interestingly, one of the main applications of the word *vulnerable* within the Oxford English Dictionary is militaristic metaphors, pointing again to the inextricably "political" dimension of illness.

8. For my own description of the phenomenology of illness, see my "Suffering, Ethics, and the Body of Christ: Anointing as a Strategic Alternative Practice," *Christian Bioethics* 2 (1996): 172–201, or my *Sharing Christ's Passion: A Critique of the Role of Suffering in the Discourse of Biomedical Ethics from the Perspective of the Theological Practice of Anointing of the Sick* (Ph.D. diss., Duke University, 1992). The phenomenology developed there is drawn primarily from three sources: Arthur Kleinman, *The Illness Narratives: Suffering and Healing in the Human Condition* (New York: Basic Books, 1998); Elaine Scarry, *The Body in Pain: The Making and Unmaking of the World* (New York: Oxford University Press, 1985); and Susan Wendell, "Toward a Feminist Theory of Disability," *Hypatia* 4 (summer 1989): 104–24. Kleinman distills his insights into patients' experiences from fifteen years' work with more than two thousand chronically ill patients and includes in that text excerpts from narratives of a number of these patients. Scarry develops an account of the "structure" of pain and its political effects drawn primarily

from accounts of persons subject to political torture—the literal inscribing of political ideology onto human bodies to solidify political power. Wendell articulates her firsthand experience of being disabled. Collectively, these three authors, and those whose observations supplement theirs, have listened to accounts of real patients or persons similarly suffering bodily affliction. These three dynamics are by no means exhaustive of the experience of illness and suffering. In light of what we will encounter in the Letter of James later, the additional factor of economic vulnerability—included in Toombs's chapter—would also usefully enhance this account.

9. H. Tristram Engelhardt Jr., *The Foundations of Bioethics* (New York: Oxford University Press, 1986), 256.

10. Kleinman, *Illness Narratives,* 16. Kleinman also poses this as a "dialogue between the voice of medicine and the voice of the life world" (129), although he clearly means that medicine dominates the conversation. See also Engelhardt, *Foundations of Bioethics,* 257.

11. Kleinman, *Illness Narratives,* 52.

12. "If there is a single experience shared by virtually all chronic pain patients it is that at some point those around them—chiefly practitioners, but also at times family members—come to question the authenticity of the patients' experience of pain." Ibid., 57; see also 59, 68. Early sufferers of AIDS and chronic fatigue syndrome experienced this denial of their claims, as medicine had not shifted their explanatory framework to include them.

13. Engelhardt, *Foundations of Bioethics,* 279.

14. Reynolds Price, *A Whole New Life: An Illness and a Healing* (New York: Plume 1995), 182–83.

15. Equally, those who reflect on suffering and illness note time and again how illness threatens the very viability of one's ideas and beliefs about how the world works. It threatens our very perception of reality, our deeply seated grasp of what is true and untrue. Such "truths," however, ought not to be understood as mentalist, disembodied constructions. Rather, the social construction of the body that illness forces us to acknowledge illuminates how "truths" are in fact embodied entities. What we find in these accounts is confirmation that through the infrastructure of social architecture, institutions, and practices, each body is inscribed by the intersection of cultural discourses of class, race, gender, age, religion, science, politics, and the individual's personal history; these intersections constitute the "code"—the truths—that provides one's ongoing identity and by which the body deciphers and negotiates the world. In instances of suffering, this embodied "code" is broken; as Art Frank notes, "In illness, the body finds itself progressively unable to express itself in conventional codes." Frank, "For a Sociology of the Body: An Analytic Review," in *The Body: Social Process and Cultural Theory,* ed. Mike Featherstone, Mike Hepworth, and Bryan S. Turner (London: Sage Publications, 1991), 85. As pain and illness grow in intensity or duration, social meanings rooted in our bodies are threatened. Illness, pain, and suffering work through the body to "dis-inscribe" it of its social meanings. They become unloosed. Scarry, *Body in Pain,* argues that the suffering of illness exerts these aversive effects more profoundly than other sorts of crises by dismantling the very substrate of social

meaning, namely, the body, and thereby dismantling what we previously held to be true about the world.

16. "Power" for Foucault is not a negative category; power is simply a necessary aspect of social existence, which functions positively or negatively. Over the past four decades, bioethics has become a corollary discourse allied with medicine in this endeavor. For example, through practices such as advance directives, biomedical ethics locates sick persons under an anthropology of autonomy, most precisely in those situations when autonomy no longer exists. For a further account of this see my "And Power Corrupts . . . : Theology and the Disciplinary Matrix of Bioethics," in *Faith at the Frontiers: A Reader in Religion and Bioethics*, ed. David Guinn (New York: Oxford University Press, 2006).

17. A third methodological commitment behind this argument can be summed up as: (3) *Lex orandi, lex credendi. As we pray, we believe. The way we know the person of Jesus Christ is through the practice of worship.* This commitment comprises three claims, one historical, one scriptural, and one philosophical. Historically, reflections on the person and work of Christ—i.e., Christology—arose as a response to the worship practices of the early church. In other words, what Christians believe theologically has always been first embodied in what they do. More precise articulations of Christian "beliefs" have always derived from reflection on practices. Although they can be separated for intellectual purposes, they cannot be separated practically. Conversely, what we do conveys what we truly believe. Some scholars have actually referred to this a "biblical epistemology." Timothy Polk, in a profound essay on Kierkegaard's surprising and appreciative championing of the Letter of James finds this biblical epistemology throughout the scripture, but particularly in James (which is quite provocative for our purposes here). As he notes,

> But appropriation demands [for Kierkegaard] that the words be put into practice; the thought must involve itself in an action. Reality being unremittingly situational, thoughts and words must get situated in the sorts of real activities that pertain to their subject matter. They must get enacted so that the relevant concepts get exercised and the reader gets capacitated in order to begin to even apprehend the reality of which the words speak. . . . [C]learly it is James' "epistemology," shared by all the biblical writers, that has shaped Kierkegaard's thinking and that he here mirrors with compelling credibility. And that biblical epistemology, never detachable from its ethics, is one in which knowing is always a function of doing, the knowledge of God always a matter of obeying God. For ancient Israel it was axiomatic that one obeyed in order to know God, while disobedience was both the sign that God had been forgotten and the means of the forgetting." (Timothy Polk, "'Heart Enough to Be Confident': Kierkegaard on Reading James," in *The Grammar of the Heart: New Essays in Moral Philosophy and Theology*, ed. Richard H. Bell [San Francisco: Harper and Row, 1988], 212–13).

Crucially, this epistemological approach admits important similarities to those proposed, in slightly different ways, by Aristotle, Foucault, and Wittgenstein. And, to highlight Polk's point, not only are practices crucial for our ability to know, but they also constitute, of course, an ethic. Thus, in sum, our practices and actions contain, embody, realize, and enact what we truly believe. Conversely, the practices in which we participate shape our beliefs, form us to believe this rather than that. To be sure, even to put it this way is somewhat problematic, insofar as the way I have phrased it suggests that practices and beliefs could be separated. But linguistic difficulties notwithstanding, this will stand as one of the fundamental claims of this chapter. Ergo, the liturgical practices of the church—how we worship—are a crucial epistemological locus for theological anthropology. What we believe about Jesus and God is inextricable from the sacraments.

18. Translations of passages from the Letter of James are taken from Luke Timothy Johnson, *The Letter of James: A New Translation with Introduction and Commentary* (New York: Doubleday/The Anchor Bible, 1995). As will become clear, the following account depends largely on Johnson's analysis, and this for two reasons: for purposes of brevity and 2 because Johnson provides one of the most thorough and compelling analyses I have found.

19. Ibid., 85. Johnson notes, "James' language is particularly shocking since, in Hellenistic moral discourse, vice and true friendship are considered to be polar opposites."

20. Ibid., 288.

21. Ibid., 85.

22. Ibid., 86.

23. James's invective against the double-minded seems particularly directed at the rich and the powerful—those who want to maintain the benefits they derive from "the world," who largely espouse the world's values (control, making money, individual prestige and power) but have, for whatever reason, affiliated themselves with James's community. In light of the position that will be developed further later, Eleanore Stumpf's claim in "Aquinas on the Sufferings of Job" is worth exploring further: "An important part of Job's suffering stems from the fact that, in the face of all the evil that has befallen him, he remains convinced not only of the existence of God but also of his power and sovereignty, and even (or perhaps especially) of his intense interest in Job. But in consequence of his sufferings Job has become uncertain or *double-minded* about the goodness of God, and so his trust in God, which had formerly been the foundation of his life, is undermined in ways that leave Job riven to his roots." Stumpf, "Aquinas on the Sufferings of Job," in *The Evidential Argument from Evil*, ed. Daniel Howard-Snyder (Bloomington: Indiana University Press, 1996), 333 (emphasis mine). James mentions Job as well, and one might suggest that James recognizes in illness the power to render us double-minded insofar as—following the Foucauldian dynamic described earlier—the worldview held by the sick can become dis-inscribed. Illness puts us in a position where the truths we held—in God's presence and beneficence—become harder to hold onto, while the truths of the world—individual competitiveness, violence as a means to my own ends (e.g., in our contemporary context, physician-assisted suicide, human embryonic stem cell research)—begin to seem more plausible and compelling. In this situation, which practices we participate in become that much more important.

24. "Let the lowly brother boast in his exalted position. But let the rich person boast in his humbling, because like a wild flower he will pass away. For the sun rises with its burning heat and dries up the grass, and its flower falls, and the beauty of its appearance is lost. Thus also the rich person will disappear in the midst of his activities." James 1:9–12.

25. "My brothers, do not hold the faith of Jesus Christ our glorious Lord together with acts of favoritism. For if a man with gold rings and splendid clothing enters your assembly, and also a poor man dressed in filthy clothing, and you look favorably on the one wearing the splendid clothing and say to him, 'you sit here in a fine place,' while you also say to the poor person, 'you stand there, or sit below my footrest,' are you not divided within yourselves [back to the double-minded], and have you not become judges with evil designs? Listen, my beloved brothers! Has not God chosen the poor in the world to be rich in faith and heirs of the kingdom which he has promised to those who love him? But you have dishonored the poor person! Is it not the rich who oppress you and are they not the very ones who are dragging you into courts? Are they not the very ones blaspheming the noble name which has been invoked over you?" James 2:1–7.

26. "Come now, you who are saying, 'Today or tomorrow we will go to a certain city and we will spend a year there and will make sales and a profit.' You are people who do not know about tomorrow, what your life will be like. For you are a mist which appears only for a moment and then disappears. Instead, you should say, 'If the Lord wills it, we will both live and do this or that thing.' But now in your pretentiousness you are boasting. Every boast of this sort is evil. Therefore it counts as a sin for the person who understand the proper thing to do and yet does not do it. Come now, you rich people! Weep and wail over the miseries that are coming to you! Your wealth has rotted, and your clothes have become moth-eaten! Your gold and your silver have rusted, and their rust will be testimony against you and will eat your flesh like fire. You have built up a treasure in the last days. Behold! The wages of the laborers who have harvested your fields—the wages of which you have defrauded them—are crying out. And the cries of the reapers have reached the ears of the Lord of Armies. You have lived luxuriously upon the earth, and you have taken your pleasure. You have stuffed your hearts for a day of slaughter. You have condemned, you have murdered the righteous one. Does [God] not oppose you?" James 4:13–5:6). James certainly is not speaking of wealth metaphorically.

27. Intriguingly, James's first elaboration of the infamous disjunction between "faith and works" concerns caring for the needy: "What use is it, my brothers, if someone says he has faith but does not have deeds? Is the faith able to save him? If a brother or sister is going naked and lacking daily food, and if one of you should say to them, 'Go in peace! Be warmed and filled,' but does not give to them what is necessary for the body, what is the use?" James 2:14–15.

28. Johnson, *Letter of James*, 81.

29. Ibid., 82.

30. Including "the self-justifying claim that one is tempted by God (1:13), the flattering speech that reveals partiality toward the rich and shames the poor (2:3–6), the superficial speech of the one claiming to have faith even without deeds (2:18) . . . judging and slandering a brother (4:11), boasting of one's future plans without

regard for God's will (4:13), and grumbling against a brother (5:9)," as well as the taking of oaths. Ibid., 255.

31. Ibid., 341.

32. Ibid., 184.

33. Ibid., 342.

34. Ibid.

35. Ibid., 343.

36. When James turns his attention to the situation of the sick, the community becomes the agent. Throughout this section, he is addressing the community: is anyone *among you* sick? Is any one *among you* ill? But even within this short space, we see a crucial difference in actions. "Is anyone among you suffering? Let *that person* pray. Is anyone feeling good? Let *that person* sing." In verse 13, individuals are exhorted to act within the community. But in the event of sickness, the dynamic shifts: "Is anyone among you sick? Let that person *call the elders of the assembly*, and *let them*, after anointing him with oil in the name of the Lord, *pray* over the person."

Interestingly, "we notice first that James empowers the sick themselves with respect to the community. When they are ill, *they* are to call the elders of the community. James's language has a formal quality: they are to *summon* the elders (5:14). James then enjoins the elders to pray over and anoint the sick person in the name of the Lord. In the elders, the *'ekklesia'* is to respond to the weak member and overcome the alienation and inertia with which sickness threatens the life of the group." Ibid., 342–43.

37. Elsewhere I have outlined how the contemporary rite of anointing of the sick responds specifically to the dynamics of illness outlined earlier. See Lysaught, "Suffering, Ethics, and the Body of Christ," 172–201, and Lysaught, *Sharing Christ's Passion*, chap. 4.

PART

4

Relationality

CHAPTER

10

Gender and Human Relationality

Christine E. Gudorf

Humans are adaptive. If we accept the theory of evolution, we understand adaptation as an aspect of all forms of life, most especially of the human species. One indication of human adaptability is our ability to live anywhere on Earth, in contrast to other animals that are limited to particular environments. This adaptability in human beings has created great cultural diversity among humans.

One central element of human adaptivity is relationality. Humans become who we are in relationship to God, to other persons, to animals, and to the environment. Morality is an aspect of our relationality—it is the quality of our response to encounters with other persons and the larger environment. The most powerful moral responses in humans are to other humans, for a number of reasons. It is other humans who make the most urgent demands on us. It is other humans who reflect back to us most clearly who we are and who we can become; they are our fullest source of knowledge of ourselves. We find it easiest to identify with other humans; such ability is the foundation of empathy, which plays a major role in moral choices and behavior.

The adaptability of humans to new situations is not a positive moral value in itself. Human adaptability has frequently ignored moral limits, which are often obscured under particular historical circumstances and only become clear in new situations characterized by greater freedom. For example, it took many centuries for human societies to recognize that slavery was not moral. Only changes in economic, social, and political circumstances allowed people to see in increasing numbers the inhumanity of owning other human beings. Today such a transformation in the status of women is slowly taking place around the world, as generation after generation of women move from situations of subjection toward situations of equality with men, due again to shifts in the economic, social, and political configurations of late modernity. One part of this shift is the gradual disappearance of polygamy as polygamy's social benefits (maximal fertility, rapid population growth, symbol of wealth and status) gradually become obscured by its incompatibilities with late modern life. In late modernity marriage becomes an exclusive relationship of interpersonal intimacy because traditional sources of intimacy disappear; children are more expensive in urban settings than they were on the farm and are dependent for longer and longer periods; and the environment can no longer sustain population growth in many areas of the world. All of these trends mitigate against polygamy.

The big debates today about sexual morality are rooted in questions about human anthropology—an understanding of human nature. There is increased agreement that the human person is not only more than simply physicality and rationality but also that the human person is relational. We have come to see that, in a broad way, human persons are constructed and that rationality is fundamental in the construction process. But there are various ways of understanding the construction process.

The Catholic natural law position has generally been understood as anticonstructionist, or at least only weakly constructionist, in that it argues for human nature as given in creation. This givenness has almost always been understood in static terms, though there have been strains—most notably in the work of Teilhard du Chardin—that have argued for dynamism as a central aspect of the human nature God created. It seems to me that the increasing shift in Catholic moral theology toward environmental consciousness is influencing natural law thought, moving it toward more openness in human nature, toward understanding adaptability, especially relationality, as central human traits that indicate/create some degree of plasticity and diversity in human nature itself.

Modern thought has had great influence on contemporary Catholic moral theology's understanding of the human person. The very term "the human person" reflects modern universalism in that it assumes there is one model, one nature for human persons. Just as feminists have rejected speech about "woman" as excluding the possibility of diversity among women, today more people are becoming uncomfortable with the concept of "the human person" and insisting on plural language that recognizes difference. We are brought to this point in part by recognition of another aspect of modern thought—developmentalism, the recognition of historical change, change that is sometimes caused by human persons, but that also changes human persons. Just as modern thought recognized changes in science, technology, and the societies they transformed, it also recognized vital changes in human persons. The church has been impacted by modern thought in a variety of ways, often adopting modern perspectives, sometimes after initial periods of resistance, and usually in gradual steps.

An example of such adoption is found in the twentieth-century papal understanding of women, their nature and role. Pius XI demanded that wives accept their honorable subjection to husbands and condemned those who falsely taught that women were equal to men, and Pius XII repeated the call for women's "sincere submission" to their husbands.[1] Pius XII and John XXIII defended women's equality with men in the eyes of God (spiritual equality) but argued that in terms of social function—certainly in marriage—women were not equal and were subject to men, though they were entitled to public as well as domestic roles if these were appropriate to their feminine nature.[2] More recently, John Paul II, in a radical rereading of the Ephesians 5:22–24 call for wives to be subject to husbands as to the Lord, has argued that the text really calls for mutual subjection of husband and wife.[3] Following his predecessor, Paul VI, John Paul II called for the full equality of men and women in the larger society as well.[4] The church's normative reading of human relationality with regard to sex has thus been transformed, at least with regard to domestic, social, and spiritual roles, if not ecclesial ones. The church still maintains that women do not resemble Christ in essential ways and thus are not able to fulfill equal functions (e.g., governance).[5] There is no explanation as to how women can be equal to men in the eyes of God, yet be so different from Christ in his maleness as to be unable to share Christ's ministerial role in the church.

Despite such clear examples of constructionism in Catholic understanding of female human nature, there are many areas of church teaching that are still strongly essentialist regarding the nature of male and female persons. While John Paul II recognized the social roles of men and women as equal, and, in society at least, as interchangeable, he maintains essentialist versions of male and female nature.[6] This is, ironically, a major shift from his predecessors, whose basic argument was that men and women were created with different and complementary natures, which were then the foundation for, and source of, the limits on men's and women's roles in family, church, and society. What has clearly happened is that the church has not been able to withstand the changes in women's transformed roles in society and has capitulated to them, forced to agree that women can perform virtually every role as well as men. One would expect that agreeing to equality and interchangeability of men's and women's social roles would imply some profound similarities in male and female natures, if nature is indeed the foundation of functional capacity. But no. John Paul II insisted on radical differences in male and female natures, that they complement one another rather than resemble each other.[7]

At another level, too, church teaching has changed regarding the relation of men and women, and that change concerns marriage. At the beginning of the twentieth century, certainly through *Casti connubii*, marriage was a contract, based not on what church—and most of society—regarded as "fleeting" affections, but on a free commitment of the will. That commitment involved the sexual gift of one's body to the spouse for purposes of reproduction, in an indissoluble bond that helped spouses avoid temptation to sexual sin. The love that developed within the ideal marriage in this model involved respect, service, fidelity, and cooperation in child rearing. Love was an obligation that accompanied the vows, not a sentiment that led persons to undertake the obligations that accompanied the vows.

Gradually, in the last half of the twentieth century, church language about marriage changed. It began to focus more on affection, on intimacy.[8] It no longer treated marital sex as something that was dangerous because its pleasure both invited excess and yet was permitted for purposes of the good of reproduction. Instead, marital sex became understood as an expression of love with the power to bind the couple together. Increasingly church documents, and certainly theologians in the church, locate the sacramentality of marriage not in reproduction, not in indissolubility or the avoidance of adultery, but in the quality of mutual love itself. This change, too, has been based in historical developments that have made sexual relationships the primary locus for interpersonal intimacy in a way that they had never been before. This change is not universal—it is a character-istic of the modern world, of urban, mobile, anonymous societies.

Unlike premodern, or even early modern societies, men and women in the late modern world have become much more alike. They have similar education and training and occupy similar occupations. Technology's har-nessing of energy has both removed the physical strength demands that reserved many jobs for men alone and lessened the reproduction and lacta-tion demands that formerly occupied most women for much of their lives, as well as removed to factories much of the domestic work that women had performed in the home while raising children. The church resisted most of these changes: Pius XI protested coeducation in particular, insisting that men and women should be trained not only separately, but differently.[9] Pius XII and John XXIII wrote often on the limited work roles that fitted women: those that replicated maternal work in the home.[10] But their voices were raised in vain.

Today the Vatican's insistence on sexual complementarity is also run-ning against the tide of history in many ways. And yet the Vatican is not alone in this essentialist insistence on complementarity. Feminists such as Luce Irigaray also argue for some essence of femaleness, and against plasticity in human sexuality, though they are not nearly as sure as John Paul II that we can say what the essence of femaleness is in a world where females are constructed without much freedom.[11] In terms of what should be done, Irigaray and other naturalist feminists are diametrically opposed to the papal understanding of action to be taken, as they argue for complete freedom for women to become "what they were meant to be" while John Paul II is arguing for limits that keep women being "what they were made to be."[12]

In many parts of the developing world, feminists insist that mother-hood is an essential aspect of women's identity, despite the occasional woman who disavows motherhood completely.[13] There is debate, of course, over whether this identity of femaleness with motherhood results from the assigned social function or precedes it. Some of these feminists see the pri-mary social bond as being between parent (especially mother) and child, as John Paul II seems to also when he speaks of motherhood,[14] whereas oth-ers see women's commitment to children as based both in an unavoidable moral imperative responding to the vulnerability of children in uncaring societies and on the exclusion of women from other social outlets for com-passion and contribution to the common good.

Neither social nor biological science has resolved these debates. While we know a great deal more about male/female differences, our increased knowledge continues to supply evidence on both sides. Biology tells us more ways in which men and women differ as groups, but also provides evidence that the range of difference within the male group overlaps to a certain extent with the range of difference within the female group on most measures. There is even evidence that some biological differences may result from functional roles rather than the reverse, as in the case of hormonal levels: a recent study showed that holding a swaddled doll for thirty minutes causes significant reductions in testosterone levels in men.[15] Similarly, the social sciences tell us how differently men and women as groups think, decide, and respond to different situations, but they also tell us that much of this difference is culturally determined and that there is, again, great overlap between the groups. One of the more interesting findings is that in civilization after civilization there is evidence that cultures exaggerate existing differences between the sexes based in biology—for example, in our own culture by socializing men to use the lower end of their biological voice range and women the higher end of their biological voice range.[16]

Patterns in relationality in our society differ by sex. In general, men individuate earlier. On many measures, the average eighteen-year-old male has the same degree of selfhood in the sense of individuation and self-identity that the average woman has in her midthirties. On the other hand, women are more inclined to have intimate relationships (usually same sex) and to form them more easily and in greater numbers. A number of researchers have dealt with various aspects of this issue. Dinnerstein, Chodorow, and Gilligan all believe that these differences—which are the basis of the major differences that most men and women point to between the sexes— are rooted in the sex of the infant caretaker, which is in our society, as in most, almost exclusively female.[17] Chodorow and Gilligan point to the infant/toddler task of reaching gender identity in the virtually exclusive company of women. Little girls use a strategy of modeling—they merely identify with and model the behavior of their caretakers, so this task rarely provokes anxiety in girls. On the other hand, because the task does not involve any discrimination, they do not receive any help in individuation, in separation from mothers and other caretakers. This is undoubtedly one reason why early adolescence is so traumatic for girls, and especially for girls' relationships with their mothers.[18] To carve out a self that is separate from that of mother is essentially a new task for girls, one in which they have no practice, but which is suddenly thrust on them at adolescence.

For boys, say Chodorow and Gilligan, the initial task of gender identity is much more anxiety ridden, because they cannot use a strategy of modeling, as they have so little access to adult males—in the United States, on average, fewer than fifteen minutes a day. Boys use a strategy of separation, pushing away from intimacy with their female caretakers in favor of independence. It is this strategy of separation that gives them their great advantage over females in identity development, but also their great disadvantage in terms of relational intimacy. Researchers who study adolescent males propose that as later tasks in the consolidation of gender identity come to the fore, many boys find separation a less than completely successful strategy and attempt to use slightly older adolescents as models of masculinity to emulate. This is one of the most common explanations for the phenomenon and structure of adolescent male gangs, based on the correlation between father absence and gang membership. Chodorow and Gilligan both call for the integration of males into early—as well as later—child care in order to force girls to learn differentiation and separation as well as modeling, and to allow boys access to adult models of masculinity.[19]

Dinnerstein points to the early connection between infants and the female body, both the connection that exists when the child is in the mother's womb and that which exists in the first months after the child is born but before he or she comprehends his or her separation from the mother's body. She posits that this early period of undifferentiation, at least from the infant's experience and perspective, is blissful.[20] The child is connected to the very source of all its desires. She or he has only to whimper or stretch to be rewarded with the comfort and care that satisfy. Dinnerstein argues that in our sexual lives men and women both try to re-create the sensual bliss we knew as infants, but that due to gender identities, we do it differently.[21] Men try to possess what they experienced as the source of bliss (a female body) while women identify with that body and seek to be desired and appreciated as that source of infant bliss.

In a more recent twist on these arguments, Eleanor Maccoby, who together with Carolyn Jacklin had published in 1974 *The Psychology of Sex Differences*,[22] an exhaustive review and analysis of existing research on sex differences in intellectual performance and behavior (of which they found very few), has published a new book that analyzes existing research on the relational patterns between the sexes.[23] Maccoby begins by looking at the interaction between the sexes in early childhood and finds that in the first two years of life, toddlers in the presence of other children do not have sexual preferences in playmates, but that in the third year they begin to demonstrate increasingly strong preferences for same sex playmates.[24] The resulting separation endures until sexual pairings begin in late adolescence, at which time both sexes are uncomfortable around the other, realizing that they do not know the ways of the other sex.[25] In families, in the workplace, and in the wider society in general, men and women often have different styles of interaction, which can be traced back to that learned in segregated childhood. Maccoby understands this difference as having a biological base as well as a socialization base. She concludes, "So, biology is not destiny. Societal gender roles are flexible. Still, certain sex-differentiating patterns of social behavior that emerge in childhood appear to have some biological roots, and have consequences for the kinds of social interactions that occur between men and women in their adult years. These childhood patterns can be seen as exercising a kind of inertial counterweight against changes in gender roles and gender relations."[26]

Where We Are Now

The tentative conclusion of research today, then, is that there are very real sex differences in which biology plays at least some part, but in which socialization and environment play at least as large, and probably a larger, part. For example, it is clear that the range of difference within each sex is far larger than the range of difference between the sexes. Interestingly, the differences that are the largest between the sexes have to do not so much with intellectual capacity or work roles, but with interpersonal relationship, especially sexual relationships and parenting roles. The two most important influences on sex roles and attitudes seem to come from two very different directions: one from the gendering of early child care, which seems to create and/or exaggerate sex differences, and the other from the late modern ungendering of society in general, as in coeducation and equal access to social roles by both sexes, which works to minimize differences.

The greater differences within a sex than between the sexes must undermine support for a purely physicalist approach to human nature when it comes to sex. And yet it would be erroneous to posit a complete plasticity to sex/gender, for even if we cannot, for example, point thus far to any specific correlations between sex of the brain and behavior, evidence of hormonal influence on behavior is fairly clear, both within and between the sexes. Both men and women experience greater interest in sex, for example, when their testosterone levels rise; among women, high estrogen levels correlate with feelings of well-being and self-confidence, and dropping estrogen levels correlate with irritability and dissatisfaction.[27]

What this means for moral theology, I suggest, is that, as scandalous as it may seem to many who are accustomed to begin moral theology with norms, we must acknowledge that we cannot speak of any definitive norms for sexual activity. Moral theology must follow human anthropology, not precede it, and we do not have clarity about sexuality within human anthropology. It simply is not clear how the current evidence correlates with Christian teaching on sex and relationality. That depends, I think, very much on *which* Christian understanding of human anthropology we are talking about, for there have been a great many shifts, even within—and perhaps especially within—modernity. It is interesting, for example, that until relatively recently in church teaching sex/gender was usually understood as peripheral to the person. The reason for this was clear—the body had a sex, but the soul did not, and the soul was the core person. This was one reason that fathers of the church such as Jerome could write that the choice of virginity made women virile and able to be saved.[28] It was women's body functions that constituted their sex; once the appetites and habits of the body were abandoned, so was sex. Augustine's explanation for the subjection of women—the sin of Eve—reflected a similar understanding, in that women could escape a large measure of subjection—and all of the pain of childbirth that constituted women's other punishment for Eve's sin—by abandoning the sexual body that Augustine saw as the base of original sin.[29] In this same vein, there were recorded, especially during and after the medieval period, lives of women who lived as men—often as active soldiers in men's clothing. While most, when discovered, were regarded as "odd," even scandalous, they were not, for the most part, regarded as denying their nature or defying the Creator. Their preference for maleness was often accepted as a rational choice.[30]

It was in the nineteenth century that early modern science began to emerge, and like modernism in general, it attempted to attribute discrete definitions to, and cause and effect for, every phenomenon. As anatomy and physiology advanced, there was a strong tendency to explain maleness and femaleness exclusively in terms of biology. Nineteenth-century physicians, for example, explained any health problem in every woman as in some way linked to her womb, even when other women were not affected. Upperclass women who suffered from tubercular flushes, weakness, and fainting, for example, were told that their wombs—not their tight corsets, restrictive dress, and lack of exercise—were the cause, even though these symptoms (especially the weakness and fainting) were not found among lower-class women who had wombs but not corsets or idleness. The extreme of this trend was the nineteenth-century phrenology craze that swept Europe and America, in which "experts" claimed to be able to "read" the intellectual and moral character of individuals by examining the shape and surface of the head.

Within Catholic theology the much earlier Thomist turn to physicalism in dealing with sexuality caused the nineteenth-century church to be open to this modern scientific attempt to base all traits and behavior in sex. The shift of the Catholic Church from Platonism to Aristotelianism, a move that was made official in 1879 when Leo XIII made Thomism the basis of all Catholic philosophy and theology,[31] did not, as might otherwise have been expected, redeem sexuality by integrating body and soul. Though Thomas had adopted Aristotle's vision of spirit/mind as integrated within materiality, his treatment of sexuality constituted the single area of exception to his general method. In sexuality he instead relied upon Ulpian's physicalism. Thus, whereas Augustine had explained women's subjection as the result of Eve's sin, Thomas concluded that Eve had little choice, for women had been created inferior from the beginning, were intended only for the work of procreation, and largely represented the animal nature in humans. Thus the area within Catholicism most open to the new scientism of modernity was the teaching on sexuality.

The result of this theological shift and complementary cultural turn was that beginning in the late nineteenth century and becoming dominant in the early twentieth century there developed in Catholic teaching a strong emphasis on sex as integral to personhood. One's sex was understood to determine one's personality and character traits, one's behavior and sexual and social roles. As we have seen, after World War II the teaching on separate social roles for men and women, on the inequality of women and the restriction of women to domestic functions, began to disintegrate, but in John Paul II we still saw insistence on sexual complementarity. John Paul II understood men and women as fundamentally different emotionally and spiritually, especially in terms of male-female relationship. Though he seems to have radically reinterpreted the traditional teaching on the headship of men in the family, rejecting it entirely, a feminist hermeneutic of suspicion requires further investigation. Certainly the institutional church as a whole has done little or nothing to include this shift of his, now more than fifteen years old, in religious education materials or in sermons or public speeches. Some feminists read this new teaching of his as parallel to a teaching of Aquinas in which he agreed with St. Paul that the body of a husband belongs to the wife and the body of the wife to the husband—but then went on to say that the nature of women was that they were naturally passive and therefore would not exercise their rights, so that discussion of rights over spousal bodies would in fact deal only with male rights over women.[32] In a similar vein, John Paul's account of the character of women is that they are naturally giving, compassionate nurturers, while men are more solitary, assertive agents. Women who might try to negotiate or insist on mutual subjection with partners can therefore be accused of violating the very feminine character to which John Paul urges them to be true. The pedestalized feminine nature that popes beginning with Pius XII have offered to women on the one hand—as more moral, compassionate, and self-sacrificial—is a trap that undermines any attempt to achieve the equality that the popes offer with the other.

It seems to me that we should reject modernity's stress on sex/gender as at the core of personhood. However, we cannot return to premodern Western understandings of sexuality. That premodern Western view understood the sexless, completely spiritual soul as the core person, who shucks off sexuality along with the body when it journeys into eternity. The body-soul dualism that underlies this premodern view is simply unacceptable today, when we understand better the extent of connection between the self and embodiment.

Certainly physical sex does not seem to be permanent in any apparent way. Reproductive capacity lasts for slightly less than half of women's lives; at about the time of menopause both men's and women's bodies begin to change, becoming more and more alike in both appearance and function, just as they were until puberty. Men lose muscle, women lose curves, and both sag. Women have lower levels of female hormones, and males lower levels of male hormones. Thus as human lives in the developed quarter of the world get longer and longer, more and more of human experience takes place in relatively ungendered stages of life. Even if we look at the profound differences between men and women that Dinnerstein, Maccoby, Gilligan, and Chodorow researched, we see that these differences lessen with age. For Chodorow and Gilligan, though men and women begin with different strengths and different agendas, they end up not all that different, because a primary task of adult women is forming a self-identity apart from their primary relationships, and a primary task of adult men is overcoming the tendency to see intimacy as a threat to gender identity, as it was in their infancy. Dinnerstein sees adult heterosexual men broadening the basis of their desire for a particular woman, moving beyond her female body as the symbol of infant bliss, and sees adult heterosexual women moving beyond sexual desire based on being desired as they desired their mother's bodies in infancy toward true desire for the joys of shared sexual partnership in the present. For Maccoby, all adult relationships between the sexes involve learning to overcome the ignorance of the other sex that developed during the years of separation and to experiment with the folkways of the other sex in fashioning a shared life.

There are also traditional sources that could be consulted as to whether sexuality penetrates to the core of the person. When Jesus responded to the trap of the Sadduccees by saying that in heaven there would be no giving or taking in marriage, did he thereby mean no one in heaven had a sex? Or that there was no sexual activity? How should we interpret the church's rejection of the teaching of Gregory of Nyssa that before original sin Adam and Eve had no genitalia, for they did not need to reproduce since they were immortal? Was the church defending sexuality as a part of original creation and thus integral to humanity? Can something like sexuality be integral to the human species, but not integral to individual human persons?

My own reading of this question is that while sexuality is a part of our biological makeup, the role it plays in human life is constructed, varying from important to relatively unimportant, depending on the individual and his/her cultural and personal environment. Sexuality is constructed partly by our biology itself: the 5 percent of persons with very low sex drives are more likely to remain unmarried, even celibate. A large part of our sexuality is determined by our religio-social culture: in a traditional culture in which the chief obligation of parents is to marry off their children by adulthood, individuals have little choice as to sexual activity, especially if they are female in patriarchal societies. And certainly some part of our sexuality is chosen by individuals themselves who negotiate or fail to negotiate with partners the sexual lifestyle and patterns that develop.

I therefore reject the argument that sex was created for love when that is read in terms of traditional natural law theory. If one argues that sex was intended by the Creator for intimate interpersonal love, one must explain why humans until very recently have been unable to discern this purpose, for certainly human history is not a record of sex being understood as made for love. Religion, civil law, literature—in all these fields the history of sex is one of women, and sometimes men, being bought and sold in marriage by fathers and husbands; of harems, polygyny, dowries, and bride-price; of brothels, pimps, and streetwalkers; of marriages made for social, political, economic, and/or military reasons, often completely independent of the principals themselves. It is a history of at least as much brutality and misogyny as it is a history of love. Clearly, sex can be an aspect of persons who are bought and sold as commodities, or it can be a commodity traded and sold by individual bodies themselves in free-will decisions, or it can be a gift of love. If human experience of sex does not provide evidence that sex was made for love, I may argue that sex has the *potential* to support or even create love, under the right circumstances, but how could I persuasively argue that it was made for love? What would count as evidence for this larger claim?

I would argue that sex *should be* for love. Our society should interpret sex as being for love not because no other interpretation is possible or morally acceptable but because such an interpretation is the most helpful in meeting basic human needs at the individual and social levels today. The conditions of late modern life have broken down traditional ties among clans, tribes, and extended families of all kinds, as well as those within traditional villages and small towns. These ties between kin and neighbors were intimate relationships that reflected back to individuals who they were. Today the breakup of these reflexive communities and the shift to mobile lifestyles in anonymous urban environments has forced people to concentrate all their intimacy demands within the nuclear family, especially on the sexual relationship. If we do not understand sex as for love, we will not cultivate intimacy in sexual relationships. We need intimacy in sexual relationships because other access to intimacy is so restricted by modern conditions. Intimacy—which is what most of us mean when we speak of marital love—must be cultivated and cared for if it is to survive. The majority of men in contemporary society admit to having no intimate relationship other than their sexual relationship—no other person to whom they feel able to tell their troubles, share their emotional joys, or admit their shortcomings—and a significant minority of women admit the same. While such a situation demonstrates the connection that now exists for many between sex and loving intimacy, it also speaks to the inadequacy of sex in representing love in our society. No one person can meet all our intimacy needs; we should have multiple sources of intimacy: kin, friendships, *and* sexual relationship.

In our particular society, and I think in late modernity in general, sexuality in the sense of maleness or femaleness is often not core material. What is core is intimacy, which in our society is conveyed most often in sexual relationships, especially for men. Many people reject postmodern doubts as to whether there is any core to human persons at all, asking whether all might be merely custom and momentary preference that can be cast off and a new person and life constructed. But it does seem to me that there is a great deal of evidence, in particular for many women, that sexuality at least, is rather plastic, even if other aspects of personhood are not. In the last generations we have much more evidence of transvestites, transgendered persons, and transsexuals than ever before. It is not clear that these are new or more common phenomena than in the past; they may just be more freely expressed in public now. But at the same time that we have evidence of significant levels of gender dysphoria, we also have what are clearly new and extensive examples of androgyny in dress, behavior, and social roles.

As sexual researchers have studied women in the last two decades, they have discovered that women's sexuality is very different from men's (which is no surprise to women!). It is more diffuse and varied in a number of different ways. Women's arousal utilizes more senses than men's. In terms of sexual orientation, both males and females show a tremendous capacity for adaptation, but women have more. Eighty percent of female homosexuals have had heterosexual relationships, and 50 percent of male homosexuals have had heterosexual relationships.[33] Among heterosexuals, about 3 percent of males and 4 percent of females have experimented with homosexual sex after puberty.[34] Female sexuality is more diffuse, diverse, and relational; females seem to respond to their particular sexual partner and to structure a sexual role for themselves in relation to that partner, while male roles are more constant. This is why we see so many more women than men move successfully from long-standing heterosexual relationships to long-standing homosexual relationships and vice versa, and why men whose sexual relationships have ended are much more likely to masturbate or pay prostitutes than are women whose relationships have ended.

Women's bodies seem to have diffuse erogenous zones, while men's erogenous zone is largely restricted to their genitalia. Many women report being sexually aroused by nursing babies, which seems inappropriate to most men, many of whom can only associate such arousal with pedophilia. Thus an argument for sexuality as being part of the core personality works much better for men than for women, as men are, at least in the present social-sexual arrangements, more narrowly relational than women. While significant numbers of women report that they fall in love with a person, not with a sex, many fewer men share this sentiment.

Though human relationality is shifting more and more to the sexual realm in people's lives in late modernity, there is some evidence that many areas of work are becoming more relational as well—with more emphasis on teamwork in a variety of fields from business to engineering. But the general trend in human life is to increasing anonymity—the replacement of village living with urban living over the last two hundred years, with economically forced mobility added on. While we interact with larger numbers of persons than our ancestors, the majority of those persons are anonymous, or at least interchangeable. We have fewer and fewer sources of reflex knowledge of ourselves, fewer sources of intimacy—and late modern culture has forced these relational functions, which used to be spread through an extended family network and lifelong neighbors and church communities, into sexual relationships. Who is the only adult who will accompany us to a new city, new job? A sexual partner—and then not always. Who do we know and trust well enough that we can accept their perspective on us as true? A sexual partner. While relationality is a capacity of human beings psychologically, the form that relationality takes in our society is in large part constructed by our economic culture, which has created densely populated cities based on the demand that labor follow jobs. Thus the cultural trend we see in late modern societies is not only the restriction of intimacy to sexual relationships but also an understanding of sexual intimacy as the key to self-knowledge and sense of selfhood, and as the glue that bonds people together. The Christian response to this trend must be nuanced. We must recognize this trend and the immensely strong pressures that create it. It is hopelessly utopian to think that most Christians can successfully resist the general trends of modernity. But Christians should not capitulate to the trend, either. This trend puts a terrible burden both on sexual relationships—for this one relationship to fill all relational needs for the partners—and on those who do not have sexual relationships, who thus often lack outlets for intimacy.

Both for celibates and for the married, the churches should stress the importance of friendship. This is traditionally a difficult emphasis for the Catholic Church in particular, which has sometimes been excessively fearful that "special friendships" among celibates may become homosexual and that outside friendships for the married may undercut loyalty to the marriage and even support adultery. It seems to me that the cost of moral suspicion regarding friendships is much too high. Both the married and the celibate need close friendships. This trend to locate intimacy in sexual relationships makes the costs of celibacy for gay and lesbian laity very, very high, higher even than for priests and religious, who presumably have a call to their vocation to balance out, at least in some small part, the costs of lack of intimacy.

Yet the present state of celibacy among priests today reflects the difficulty of bucking the trend for intimacy in modernity, as do the rates of clerical alcoholism and mental disturbance, especially depression.

In thinking about relationality and sex/gender, my recommendation is twofold: I believe that society should recognize and accept/return to the decentering of sex/gender as core aspects of personhood and support sexual relationships as important but not exclusive avenues to intimacy and bonding, without establishing either of these directions as either "natural" or morally necessary. Relationality and sexuality are both "natural" for humans, but the directions that they take are constructed within a historical process and change over time. Because such changes are largely unavoidable, no particular form can be morally necessary. This does not mean that all forms are equally moral. Some forms of sex/gender interaction and of relationality are less moral than others, and some are clearly immoral. Respect for human dignity, love of neighbor, equality of persons—these criteria determine the morality of various forms of relationship.

Late modern culture is destroying relational habitats, to the extreme detriment of humaneness. The influences of a capitalist economy built on obsolescence are clear—we have throw-away families, throw-away marriages, throw-away friendships. People are as disposable as TV dinners, razors, or pens. Those relationships we don't see thrown away we see traded in, like a new car, house, or computer. Relationships must be defended by the Christian churches. The most available immediate fortress is sexual relationship, because that is where we find most of the individuals who have been successful in fending off capitulation to an anonymous society of relationless automatons with no sense of self. But the fortresses of sexual relationship are insufficient to protect society as a whole. Intimacy sufficient to support our growth and reveal us to ourselves requires the development and cherishing of friendships too.

Applications of these two suggestions in bioethics are more difficult. The recognition that sex/gender is not so central to personhood as we had thought in late modernity should give us great pause concerning transsexualism. If sex/gender is not so central to personhood then there is little imperative to do radical surgery to alter persons' sex, especially since sex/gender often transitions. On the other hand, sex/gender seems more central to males, who are less able/open to transitions. New feminist understandings of the body as inscribed might support surgical flexibility but also might conclude that the social power to inscribe makes surgical inscription unnecessary or futile, depending on whether the surgical intention supports or opposes dominant social forces. Thus the argument for the necessity of transsexual surgery is weakened, but the arguments against it are also weakened by the decentering of sex/gender from the core person.

The de-centering of sex/gender can also support intersexuality and lead to increased opposition to surgical interventions in sexually ambiguous children who have already achieved gender identity. These children have for many decades now been surgically altered to fit the sex of gender-identity rather than the chromosomal sex. Organizations such as the Intersex Society of North America have argued against surgical imposition of the dimorphic sexual paradigm, and for the legitimacy of intersexuality.[35]

In addition to these very specific influences, de-centering sex/gender might well change the terms used and the categories chosen for research in bioethics more than it will alter treatments offered. While it is difficult to imagine a time when medical charts did not routinely describe patients as male or female, we have already come to the point where many parts of the health care system do not, as they did in the past, note homosexual orientation on medical charts. It is not too difficult to imagine a future in which doctors, and the questions in medical histories, do not assume heterosexuality as the unmarked marker. Already many areas of medicine, notably professionals working with HIV/AIDS and other sexually transmitted diseases, are clear that labels—heterosexual, homosexual, married, single—are ambiguous indicators of behavior. Sexually active/inactive, number of partners, and use or nonuse of condoms in sex are much more pertinent and do not denote sex or orientation.

Prioritizing sexual/reproductive (kin) relationships does not necessarily maximize human welfare. One of my sons spent most of August and September in the intensive care unit (ICU). His father and youngest brother and I were only able to visit him twice during that time because he was 1,100 miles away. But we could not get permission from the hospital for his health care aide, who has been taking care of him for five years and is a close friend, or his oldest friend from grade and high school, who roomed with him through college, to visit. They were routinely turned away as not "family." Nor was any attempt made to ask the patient himself if he wished to receive the visitors, even after he was fully conscious. In many hospitals, patients are routinely counseled to name kin as health care surrogates, even when they are either not near and/or not close to the patient. But sometimes our children are the least able to make these quality of life and death decisions for us because they are conflicted either by their own unfulfilled needs or guilt or ignorance of us as persons. If more of us appointed health care surrogates based on honest consideration of who understands our wishes the best, the result would be less pressure to name next of kin and more openness to naming a prioritized list of close friends. Hospitals should follow suit by using such lists not only for decision making but also for visiting access.

Last, and perhaps most importantly, medical and psychological personnel who work in counseling young people need to be less focused on sexual labels and definitions. Instead of trying to categorize people into the appropriate boxes of sex/gender and orientation, they need to assure often desperately worried youth that their sexual interactions have a dynamic element in them. It simply is not true that heterosexual persons of a certain sex "inherit" a given structure for self that other persons need to construct from scratch. Whether we like it or not, for many youth today heterosexuality has more and more elements of choice and discernment. Sex/gender/ orientation are not always central to our core self. Sexual interactions are not completely plastic, but neither are they cast in stone. The kind of sexual relationship that seems right at the moment may not indicate a permanent direction. What youth should concentrate on is the quality of the relationship, and not its category. Do their relationships have a positive influence on the growth and development of both partners, whether those relationships are friendships or sexual relationships? So long as ambiguity is present, the relationship should not progress toward degrees of sexual intimacy that may imply promises that cannot be kept, either because one partner will transition sex/gender or because one partner will opt for a different sexual orientation. Once vows have been made to a partner, those vows should be kept unless one partner releases the other from them. Sexuality, like life, can be messy and somewhat ambiguous. The assumption that discovering that one is "really" male or female, gay or straight, will make one's life journey clear can simply be a terrible hoax, a remnant of the pseudoscience that gave us phrenology.

Young people increasingly intuit today that sexual pleasure is one important kind of glue in sexual relationships, that it is not only an expression of already existing love but a re-creation, and sometimes an expansion, of that already existing love. People increasingly recognize that procreation should not be the intention for sex—that sexual acts open to procreation must be rarer and rarer today. Instead, the future potential for procreation, or the already realized procreative potential in sex, should be celebrated in every sexual act. And it often is. When I make love with my husband of thirty-seven years, I make love to the young teenager I fell in love with, to the tender new father who held his child in wonder, as well as the strong adult man who occasionally rages at the need to help his child prepare for death. And that lovemaking is intimately tied to the growth in both of us that has carried us through these stages.

NOTES

1. Pius XI, *Casti connubii*, AAS 22 (1930): no. 74; *Divini Redemptoris*, AAS 29 (1937): no. 71; Pius XII, *Atti e Discorsi di Pio XII* 3 (1942): 231.

2. Christine E. Gudorf, *Catholic Social Teaching on Liberation Themes* (Washington, DC: University Press of America, 1980), chap. 5; John XXIII, *Ad Petri cathedram*, AAS 51 (1959): 509.

3. John Paul II, *Mulieris dignitatem*, AAS 43 (1988): no. 10.

4. Paul VI, *Ricordi antichi*, Osservatore Romano, December 8, 1974.

5. Congregation for the Doctrine of the Faith, *Inter Insigniores (Declaration on the Question of the Admission of Women to the Ministerial Priesthood)*, in *Women Priests: A Catholic Commentary on the Vatican Declaration*, ed. Leonard and Arlene Swidler (Mahwah, NJ: Paulist Press, 1977), 353. Also Paul VI, *Ministeria quaedam*, AAS 64 (1972): 530.

6. See Christine E. Gudorf, "Encountering the Other: The Modern Papacy on Women," *Social Compass: International Review of Sociology of Religion* 36, no. 3 (1989): 295–310.

7. For example, John Paul II, "Parati semper," *The Pope Speaks* 30 (1985): 210.

8. By intimacy, I mean a mutual knowledge and acceptance of the other that includes emotional knowledge and acceptance. Within an intimate relationship, one's hopes, fears, dreams, guilts, and insecurities can be disclosed with trust. This is both a deeper and a broader intimacy than genital intimacy alone, but it need not include genital intimacy. Many women in developed nations, for example, have more intimate relationships with close women friends than with their spouse, in the sense of freedom of emotional disclosure and mutuality of disclosure, yet these relationships are entirely nongenital. Some men have such intimacy in nongenital relationships with other men, though male-male nonhomosexual relationships in Euro-American culture (but not in some other world cultures) tend to be based in shared activities (sports, work) rather than shared feelings.

9. Pius XI, *A Lei, Vicario Nostro*, AAS 20 (1928): 136–37.

10. Pius XII, *Le vingt-cinquieme, Atti e Discorsi di Pio XII* 3 (1941): 261; "Address to Italian Women, October 21, 1945," AAS 37 (1945): 291–93; "Radio Message to the Federation of Italian Women," AAS 48 (1956): 785.

11. At the same time, Irigaray recognizes that such freedom is problematic, in that women have not only been captives of historical patriarchy but are trapped in a doubleness, a colonized situation, by their own relationality. Luce Irigaray, "This Sex Which Is Not One," in *Writing on the Body: Female Embodiment and Feminist Theory*, ed. Katie Conboy, Nadia Medina, and Sarah Stanbury (New York: Columbia University Press, 1997), 248–56.

12. John Paul II, *Laborem exercens, AAS* 73, no. 19 (1982): 107–9; "Mary Hope of all Generations," *The Pope Speaks* 24 (1979): 366–70; "Chi Triamo," *The Pope Speaks* 24 (1979): 166; "All'Indirizzo," *The Pope Speaks* 24 (1979): 181–82.

13. See, for example, Elizabeth Amoah and Mercy Amba Oduyoye, "The Christ for African Women," in *With Passion and Compassion: Third World Women Doing Theology,* ed. Virginia Fabella and Mercy Amba Oduyoye (Maryknoll, NY: Orbis Books, 1988), 45; Marianne Katoppo, *Compassionate and Free: An Asian Woman's Theology* (Maryknoll, NY: Orbis Books, 1979), 83; Jean Said Makdisi, "The Mythology of Modernity," in *Feminism and Islam: Legal and Literary Perspectives,* ed. Mai Yamani (New York: New York University Press, 1996), 248.

14. John Paul II, *Mulieris dignitatem, AAS* 79 (1988): no. 18.

15. A. E. Storey, C. L. Walsh, R. L. Quinton, and K. E. Wynne-Edward, "Hormonal Correlates of Paternal Responsiveness in New and Expectant Fathers," *Evolution and Human Behavior* 21(2000): 79–95.

16. Nancy Henley and Barry Thorne, "Womanspeak and Manspeak: Sex Differences and Sexism in Communication, Verbal and Nonverbal," in *Beyond Sex Roles,* ed. Alice G. Sargent (St. Paul: West Publishing, 1977), 201–18.

17. Nancy Chodorow, *The Reproduction of Mothering* (Berkeley: University of California Press, 1979), and Carol Gilligan, *In a Different Voice: Psychological Theory and Women's Development* (Cambridge, MA: Harvard University Press, 1982).

18. Mary Pipher, *Reviving Ophelia: Saving the Selves of Adolescent Girls* (New York: G. P. Putnam's Sons, 1994).

19. Chodorow, *Reproduction of Mothering,* 173–220; Gilligan, *In a Different Voice,* 7–11, 171.

20. Dorothy Dinnerstein, *The Mermaid and the Minotaur: Sexual Arrangements and Human Malaise* (1977; repr., New York: HarperPerennial, 1991).

21. Ibid.

22. Eleanor Emmons Maccoby and Carolyn Jacklin, *The Psychology of Sex Differences* (Stanford, CA: Stanford University Press, 1974).

23. Eleanor E. Maccoby, *The Two Sexes: Growing Up Apart, Coming Together* (Cambridge, MA: Harvard University Press, 1998).

24. Ibid., 32.

25. Ibid., 196–201.

26. Ibid., 305.

27. Tina S. Miracle, Andrew W. Miracle, and Roy F. Baumeister, *Human Sexuality* (Upper Saddle River, NJ: Prentice Hall, 2003), 84.

28. Rosemary R. Ruether, "Virginal Feminism in the Fathers of the Church," in *Religion and Sexism,* ed. Rosemary R. Ruether (New York: Simon and Schuster, 1974), 161, 175–76.

29. Ibid., 158.

30. Gilbert Herdt, *Same Sex, Different Cultures: Exploring Gay and Lesbian Lives* (Boulder, CO: Westview Press, 1997), 102–6.

31. Leo XIII, *Aeterni patris,* August 4, 1879, *Acta Sanctae Sedis* 12:97–115.

32. Thomas Aquinas, *Summa Theologiae Suppl.,* 42, as quoted in Eleanor Como Mclaughlin, "Women in Medieval Theology," in *Religion and Sexism,* ed. Ruether.

33. R. C. Savin-Williams and R. E. Lenhart, "AIDS Prevention among Gay and Lesbian Youth: Psychosocial Stress and Health Care Intervention Guidelines," in *Behavioral Aspects of AIDS*, ed. D. G. Ostrow (New York: Plenum, 1990), 75–99; R. C. Savin-Williams, "Dating and Romantic Relationships among Gay, Lesbian and Bisexual Youth," in *The Lives of Lesbians, Gays and Bisexuals: Children to Adults*, ed. R. C. Savin-Williams and K. C. Cohen (Orlando, FL: College Publishers, 1996), 166–80; M. Rosario, H. F. L. Meyey-Bahlberg, J. Hunter, and T. M. Exner, "The Psychological Development of Urban Lesbian, Gay and Bisexual Youths," *Journal of Sex Research* 33 (1996): 113–26.

34. R. T. Michael, E. O. Gagnon, and G. Kolata, *Sex in America* (Boston: Little, Brown, 1994), 176.

35. Karen Lebacqz, "Difference or Defect? Intersexuality and the Politics of Difference," *The Annual of the Society of Christian Ethics* 17 (1997): 213–29.

Bioethics, Relationships, and Participation in the Common Good

Lisa Sowle Cahill

Relationality is so integral a dimension of being human that it would be impossible to define morality without it. It is thus essential to any view of the human that could successfully ground a theologically informed bioethics. In fact, a recent publication of the Catholic Health Association (CHA) begins a discussion of relationality with this statement: "Human beings are made in the image of a triune God whose very nature is to be in relationship. As such, we are relational or social by nature. We are meant to exist in relationships—with ourselves, with others, with the rest of creation, and with God. Our flourishing as human beings only occurs in the context of relationships. And our fulfillment, our destiny, consists in relationship—communion with God."[1]

I doubt that anyone would disagree with this statement, and that is perhaps the only difficulty in taking relationality as a foundation of a theological anthropology for bioethics. It would be easy to keep our discussion at the level of platitudes. There are, however, hard questions that follow from the fact of human relationality.

It is human to be in relationships—but what kind of relationships are we in? What is their moral quality? Is relationship essentially benign and cooperative, or is it inherently competitive and conflictual? Even if it is cooperative, is it possible to meet all the requirements and obligations of relationality successfully, at all times and in relation to all persons? Isn't the reality of conflicting values, relationships, and roles of the essence of morality too? And who defines proper relationship, or the best way to set priorities and resolve conflicts?

Does a *theological* anthropology provide insights that a philosophical or political perspective cannot? Is theological bioethics based on a special view of the human, and an understanding of relationality that will put us at odds with broader views of virtue, justice, social ethics, public policy, and the good society? Are we theological bioethicists ultimately talking to ourselves?

And even if we can come to agreement with others on the basic meaning of the human as relational, and the basic shape of a good society, what makes us think that that vision can be achieved in practice? Is a Christian anthropology, especially in its Catholic "common good" versions, hopelessly naïve about the social and political realities that, for example, are causing 45 million people to be without health insurance in this country, or 44 million worldwide to be victims of AIDS?

My purpose here is to make the case that a Christian view of human relationality converges with a very basic human experience—interdependence with others in community. There is in fact some common ground in talking about the good society, and about what justice means in bioethics. While acknowledging the reality of competition and conflict, I propose that there is an equal, if not greater, human drive toward cooperation. Religious narratives and symbols can be powerful agents in evoking inclusion and cooperation as moral values and aims.

Finally, I argue that the Catholic common good tradition must verify its claims by doing more than talking about ideals; it must combat pessimism and "moral realism" by showing how those ideals can be, and are being, put into practice. As examples, I will use, first, the actual practice of Catholic health services as an institutional response to the need for justice in health care access in this country, and second, the response of transnational Catholic organizations and networks to the AIDS crisis. It is not easy to make a credible and nonnative case for a positive, confident, activist, and social transformationist approach to relationality as a basis for theological bioethics. As Reinhold Niebuhr famously remarked, original sin is the only Christian doctrine for which there is empirical verification. But I propose to show that Christian (Catholic) bioethics can reform relationships of health care, and offer at least some empirical verification of the doctrine of redemption, by advancing the potential for human relationships to be healed.

My argument consists of four parts: (1) relationality and responsibility, to use the moral language of H. Richard Niebuhr; (2) biblical resources, especially the "image of God" and "the preferential option for the poor"; (3) Catholic social tradition, with its emphases on the sociality of the person, the common good, participation, and solidarity; and (4) the relationship of a theoretical anthropology of relationality to social practices that realize relationality in a practical and challenging way.

Relationality and Responsibility

I pair relationality with responsibility in order to lift up the moral question as a disputed question. As I mentioned, few would disagree that humans, like all other beings, are relational. The mere fact that we occupy a physical environment with other creatures is enough to guarantee that. But what is the quality of our relationships? What kinds of relationships are "natural" to human beings? As Plato, Aristotle, Aquinas, and other great thinkers have taught, human beings are distinguished by the characteristics of intellect and will. Although every creature has relationships to its environment, human beings make decisions about what kinds of relationships those will be. This is not just a Catholic idea, or even a uniquely Christian one.

The Protestant theological ethicist H. Richard Niebuhr expressed the human quality of relationships in the experiential language of "responsibility." Responsibility captures "the idea of an agent's action as response to an action upon him [or her] in accordance with his interpretation of the latter action and with his expectation of response to his response; and all of this in a continuing community of agents."[2] Human relationality is, then, historical, dynamic, and interactive. It is also communal. Niebuhr sorts responsibility into four parts: *response* to actions upon us, to which we continually reply; *interpretation*, as we raise the prior question "What is going on?"; *accountability*, which means we act in anticipation of reply;

and *social solidarity*, for our actions and interactions form a continuing society.[3]

Response is then the inner moral dimension of relationality, and *responsibility* is a word that defines the moral character of responsive relationships. To act responsibly is to act accountably and in a spirit of social solidarity, as we interpret our environment and interact with our fellow human beings, and for that matter, with the whole of creation. Not all response is responsible; some moral interactions are vicious, violent, selfish, and destructive. But responsibility defines in a general way the positive moral meaning of relationality that anchors the vision of theological bioethics. The ideal of responsibility also gives Christian theological bioethics a language of discourse that is grounded in experience and can be shared with other faith traditions, other cultures, and philosophical ethics. Now we must begin to specify what responsibility means.

Biblical Resources

The idea that humans are made in the "image of God" is a keynote for the special character of humanity for Jewish and Christian traditions. To act responsibly in our relationships is to honor the image of God reflected in us. In the first creation story in Genesis, God surveys the Earth and the creatures God has made, and says,

> Let us make humankind in our image, according to our likeness; and let them have dominion over the fish of the sea, and over the birds of the air, and over the cattle, and over all the wild animals of the earth, and over every creeping thing that creeps upon the earth.
> So God created humankind in his image,
> In the image of God he created them;
> Male and female he created them.
> God blessed them. (Genesis 1:26–28)

In the history of interpretation of this passage, there has been a tendency to see it as underwriting the dignity of the unique individual, especially as rational, and to focus on the male-female relationship as part of the image, whether to argue that sexual differentiation is essential to humanity or to argue that both sexes are created equally in God's image. I take interpretation of this passage in a somewhat different direction. I emphasize *relationality* as essential to God's image and present the creation of male and female as the first instance of human relationship. The image of God is more significant because of the fact that it establishes basic human relationality than because it establishes sex or gender relationships.

In a work on stewardship commissioned by the National Council of Churches, Douglas John Hall links the image of God in humanity with relationality. God intends humanity to be a "being-in-relationship." Humanity's essential nature is not found in the abstract or in an isolated specimen defined by certain capacities, but "by considering human beings in the context of their many-dimensioned relationships."[4] The distinctive characteristics of humans, such as intellect and will, exist only for the purpose of entering into relationships with others and with God.[5]

Biblical scholars, especially Claus Westermann, have confirmed this idea that the image of God must be sought in relationship.[6] The image has an essentially social meaning. The norm of human community established by the biblical symbol image of God is a social unity-in-difference. This is revealed by the immediate differentiation of humanity into "others" who are essentially of the same nature and equally reflective of the divine. Sexual differentiation and relationship exemplify the relationality of the human per se. Humans, as constitutively different from one another, are also constitutively destined for relationship; the same holds true for human groups or societies. Being in relational groups, from the sexual pair to the family to the local community to the region, nation, continent, and globe—this is what it means to be made "in the image of God."

The *quality* of relationship is another issue. If human relationships are to image God's relationships, then they are certainly to be just and even loving. As Hall maintains, humans are called to *hesed* or, in New Testament terms, *agape*.[7] Unfortunately, and too familiarly, love is not the purpose to which the "image of God" is customarily put. Christians in practice often have picked up on the "dominion" theme of Genesis, granting humans the license to exploit the rest of creation, men to dominate women, and supposedly "Christian" cultures to colonize and exploit other groups deemed not to reflect God's image or not to reflect it in the same way or to the same extent.[8]

The sinful human tendency to dominate vulnerable persons and groups was challenged eloquently by the Hebrew prophets, especially Amos, Hosea, and Isaiah. Amos, for example, bases his demand for justice and care for the outcast and oppressed on his conviction that God rules the world and holds Israel especially responsible for a righteous way of life.

This responsibility has been betrayed by those who "sell the just person for money and the poor for a pair of shoes, and trample the heads of the impoverished into the dust of the ground and shove the afflicted aside on the road" (2:6–7). Isaiah quotes the Lord as saying, "What do you mean by crushing my people, by grinding down the faces of the poor?" (3:15).

In Luke's gospel, the ministry of Jesus is inaugurated in his hometown when he reads in the temple from the scroll of Isaiah: "The Spirit of the Lord is upon me, because he has anointed me to bring glad tidings to the poor . . . to let the oppressed go free" (4:18). The mission and ministry of Jesus can be seen, in their moral dimensions, to consist of a challenge to human relationships disordered by abuse of power and of a redefinition of proper relationship to others and to God as informed by love and inclusion, and by actions that express such relationships. The focal symbol of Jesus's ministry, "reign of God" (Mark 1:14), is comprised by a call to repentance and to a reversal of ordinary power relationships, in which the strong exploit the weak. The parable of judgment in Matthew 25 applies very well to responsibility to seek the physical and spiritual well-being of our fellow humans, a responsibility that is foundational for health care. The deeds to which Jesus' disciples are called are to feed the hungry, give drink to the thirsty, welcome the stranger, clothe the naked, and visit the imprisoned. These actions express relations of respect, inclusiveness, altruism, and mercy. The parable also illustrates the close connection between human relationships and humanity's relation to God. "Come," says Jesus, "you that are blessed by my Father" (Matt. 25:34). "Truly I tell you, just as you did it for one of the least of these who are my family, you did it for me" (Matt. 25:40).

The symbol of "family" reveals the types of relationships to which we are called. Jesus, of course, is not referring to families of blood or marriage but to the new, inclusive community constituted in his name. This new family in Christ cuts across boundaries of sex, race, class, and religion (Gal. 3:28), and of blood relationship as well. It is open to all who are willing to hear the word of God and do it (Mark 3:34–35; Luke 11:27–28). We are newly born as brothers and sisters in Christ, into a family that can also be imaged as the "body of Christ" (1 Cor. 10:16–17). The image of the community as Christ's body not only conveys that it represents the sort of redeemed relationships that authentically represent Christ in this world but also gives texture to the real, embodied, and concrete nature of human relationality. *Responsibility* in relationship calls us to practical works and actions on behalf of our fellow human beings, and to creation of new practices, patterns, and institutions that structure human relationships differently, both locally and globally. Relationality in New Testament perspective requires that we who are privileged make what liberation theologians and John Paul II have called a "preferential option for the poor."[9]

The intrinsic relationality of God and humanity is a fundamental theme in the entire theological tradition, and especially in the creedal and conciliar formulations of God as triune and as related to humanity in Christ. According to Catherine LaCugna, "The point of Trinitarian theology is to convey that it is the essence or heart of God to be in relationship to other persons; that there is no room for division or inequality or hierarchy in God; that the personal reality of God is the highest possible expression of love and freedom; that the mystery of divine life is characterized by self-giving and self-receiving; that divine life is dynamic and fecund, not static or barren."[10] The Christian community is called to "be an icon" of the trinitarian life of God; the Christian person is called to participate in the divine life by living in conformity to Jesus Christ by the power of the spirit. This requires that Christian persons and the church change patterns of human relationships toward greater reciprocity and participation.[11]

Catholic Social Tradition

Beginning with Leo XIII's *Rerum novarum* in 1891,[12] recent Catholic social teaching, including the modern papal social encyclicals, the documents of the Second Vatican Council, theological writings in social ethics, political and liberation theology, and many statements and addresses of John Paul II, have upheld the sociality of the person and taken its moral requirements into national, international, and global society. Though inspired by biblical and gospel ideals, responsible human relationality is viewed in this tradition as a natural capacity of humans and societies, one that is distorted by willful wickedness but remains intact enough to fund common discourse about what morality and justice demand.

A key category, defining justice and responsibility as the meanings of relationality, is the common good. The Second Vatican Council defines the common good as "the sum of those conditions of social life which allow social groups and their individual members relatively thorough and ready access to their own fulfillment."[13] The dignity of every person, and the interdependence and social participation of all, structure the responsible relationality that make up the common good. In this tradition, the dignity of the person and the common good are interdependent and complementary. Individual rights are paired with duties, both in the sense that persons have duties to ensure that the civil and material rights of all are met and in the sense that rights exist as the conditions necessary for all to fulfill their duties to the common good. The reconciliation of rights and duties, and the mediation of conflict, are the duties of the civil government, existing on many levels from local to national to international.

As *Gaudium et spes* observes, "Every day human interdependence grows more tightly drawn and spreads by degrees over the whole world."[14] As a result, the meaning of the common good has become increasingly comprehensive. Vatican II and John XXIII, Paul VI, and John Paul II have increasingly posed the responsibilities demanded by the common good in universal terms.[15] Paul VI and John Paul II, in the strongest possible words, make the case that responsibility to the universal common good requires the personal and social virtue of solidarity. Responsibility and solidarity require the actual redistribution of economic and social resources, so that the wealthy neither profit by the misery of the poor nor stand by while other human beings and societies suffer lack of basic needs.[16] For John Paul II, the recognition of interdependence demands a correlative response: a "moral and social attitude," which, "'as a virtue,' is *solidarity*." Solidarity is not a vague feeling of compassion, but "a *firm and persevering determination* to commit oneself to the *common good*; that is to say to the good of all and of each individual, because we are all really responsible *for all*."[17]

As a social virtue, solidarity requires institutions and structures. Social practices provide consistency and stability, furnish a mechanism for cooperation, and make it possible to mediate compassionate and solidaristic action from one group or locale to another that may be distant in place or time. According to the "principle of subsidiarity,"[18] local relationships should be governed at the local level, where concrete needs and obligations can be more accurately specified and more cooperatively met. However, more comprehensive or inclusive authorities have the responsibility to intervene when necessary to ensure that all are able to contribute to, and benefit from, the common good.[19]

John Paul II notes a novel development in the modern world—the active participation of the world's disenfranchised in taking action for social change. "Positive signs in the contemporary world are the growing awareness of the solidarity of the poor among themselves, their efforts to support one another," and their resistance to "the inefficiency or corruption of the public authorities."[20] To this one must also add the apathy, bad faith, and outright manipulation of powerful countries, classes, and corporations. However, by and large, Catholic social tradition is only gradually moving from the hierarchical and organic model of society assumed by the earliest encyclicals toward the realization that the interests of different social groups might be very hard to harmonize. The will of the powerful to initiate change may be totally lacking, the empowerment of the marginalized essential, and the coercion of their adversaries, either by law or by some sort of revolution, are absolutely required if change is to occur.

The principle of subsidiarity needs to be reinvigorated and renegotiated in this regard. It should refer not just to an orderly, vertical delegation of authority from higher to lower groups arranged like concentric circles but also to morally authoritative action initiated outside the formally legitimated structures of authority, and to horizontal, midlevel, pluralistic, and intersecting energies and forces that challenge the status quo and create new networks and alliances that can be effective for change.

Relationality, Responsibility, and Practical Theological Bioethics

Papal, episcopal, and theological writings on health care all confirm that responsibility in the relations that constitute the common good demands a "preferential option for the poor" in health care, and structural justice that ensures access for all. For instance, the U.S. Catholic bishops in their landmark "Resolution on Health Care Reform," assert that "every person has a right to health care. This right flows from the sanctity of human life and the dignity that belongs to all human persons, who are made in the image of God." Moving to social responsibility, they invoke "the biblical call to heal the sick and to serve 'the least of these,' the priorities of social justice and the common good," the "virtue of solidarity," and "the option for the poor and vulnerable."[21]

The "Resolution on Health Care Reform" was published more than a decade ago, at the time of the failed attempt of President Bill Clinton to put health care reform on the national agenda in a meaningful way. Despite the bishops' interventions, and those of many theological bioethicists, we are now worse off than we were at that time. There has been some expansion of Medicare, and the institution of a federal- and state-funded health insurance program for children (SCHIP, in 1997). However the U.S. Census Bureau reports that the number of uninsured continues to rise, more than 45 million at last count.[22]

Globally, many more persons than that lack access to what most Americans would consider "adequate" health care, or even the basic conditions of a safe and healthy life, such as food, clean water, and protection from violence. The "diseases of the poor," such as AIDS, malaria, and tuberculosis, plague millions. When the fifteenth International AIDS Conference met in Bangkok in July 2004, 40 million people worldwide were infected with that disease alone. Yet in 1990, long before most world leaders were aware of and invested in the crisis, John Paul II warned that "AIDS threatens not just some nations or societies but the whole of humanity. It knows no frontiers of geography, race, age or social condition. The threat is so great, indifference on the part of public authorities, condemnatory or discriminatory practices toward those affected by the virus or self-interested rivalries in the search for a medical answer, should be considered forms of collaboration in this terrible evil which has come upon humanity."[23] In a statement to the United Nations more than a decade later, a Vatican official was still hammering home the point that "extreme poverty experienced by a great part of humanity" is a key cause of AIDS, making it an urgent matter of "international social justice."[24]

Is any of this making a difference? Are we theological bioethicists forced to draw the conclusion that talk about responsible relationality in Catholic bioethics is just that—talk? My answer is that theological "talk" is important because it clarifies the coherence and implications of our religious beliefs and practices. It can also draw connections between our traditions and theologies and the worldviews and practices of other traditions, both religious and nonreligious. But ultimately, especially when we are talking about theological *ethics*, the theory (theology or "talk) has a practical flip side. The present volume on a "theological anthropology" for bioethics is very much rooted in practical concerns, which would be evident if for no other reason than the fact that it is being sponsored by a center for *clinical* bioethics.

It is not only that practice stimulates theoretical reflection and shapes its direction and content, though that of course is true. Theological ethics, including bioethics, also engages with practices, approaches practices critically and constructively, and is validated in its content and truth by the sort of practices it inspires. Although the "anthropological" premises of Christian-Catholic theological bioethics may not have converted worldwide structures of access to the goods of health, theological bioethics does operate in tandem with institutional practices that are challenging these structures and serving as catalysts for change.

I offer two examples. The first is the engagement of Catholic health services and their professional organization, the Catholic Hospital Association, with the problem of inequitable health care access in this country. The second is the engagement of Catholic transnational agencies and networks with the AIDS crisis. I will focus on one example, a project by women's religious congregations to empower women in Africa against the plague of HIV infection.

Catholic Health Association and Catholic Health Care

If we look at national health policy, it may seem that the bishops and theologians have made little impact. However, taking our cue from recent studies of "civil society," "participatory democracy," and so on, it is equally important to look at what is happening "on the ground."[25] Catholic health care is not a negligible place to look for wide-reaching practices of social change. Today two thousand Catholic health care sponsors, systems, facilities, and related organizations serve across the continuum of care; one in six Americans is cared for in a Catholic acute care facility; and the Catholic health ministry is the largest not-for-profit provider of health services in the nation.[26]

This ministry goes beyond providing charity care in a broken system, however. Drawing on theological and ethical scholarship, on a historical tradition of service to the poor, and on contemporary principles of social justice and the common good, the CHA has made advocacy for structural transformation in law, policy, and practice a major priority. Its website provides links to church teaching, position papers, policy status reports, health facility and systemwide initiatives, and advocacy opportunities too numerous to mention. In 2000, the CHA Board of Trustees approved *Continuing the Commitment: A Pathway to Health Care Reform* to establish a vision for a Catholic reform initiative.[27] Citing its history of crafting policy proposals and of fostering grassroots advocacy, the CHA planned to wage a national battle to put incremental extensions of coverage as well as global policy changes on the agendas of caregivers, legislators, faith communities, and the general public. The CHA's position is that all persons living in this country should be entitled to a package of basic services and that a supplemental package should be available for purchase.

Catholic health care providers, scholars, and leaders, demonstrating "bioethics in action," are not waiting for change from the federal government. On the basis of subsidiarity, they take the initiative in devising more just and inclusive approaches to care, approaches that not only serve but aim to empower the underserved and their communities. For example, in a report on "Catholic Ministries as Catalysts for Healthier Communities," the CHA offers standards, software, publications, meetings, and continuing groups and networks.[28] The goal is to enhance collaborative efforts among religious, nonprofit, governmental, and health care institutions to support preventive services, basic care, and community support for those suffering chronic illness. The CHA has similar initiatives for the dying and the elderly, and in all cases health care as such is linked with other social goods and services, such as housing.

The presidential election year 2004 put health care reform on the national agenda once again. The mandate of Catholic social teaching is clear: universal access. Distributive justice defines relational responsibility in health care. Catholic health care leaders advocate for top-level governmental leadership, financing, and intervention on behalf of equitable health care for all. But as ethics "on the ground," Catholic theological bioethics has also begun to institutionalize patterns of action that, imbued with the virtue of solidarity, are putting into practice responsible relationships around the goods of health care, relationships that are already beginning to transform at the local level.

AIDS and Globally Responsible Relationships

At a 2004 news conference marking the pope's Lenten message on behalf of children, the Vatican called on Catholic leaders to fund the campaign against AIDS. It announced its own efforts, by means of the issuing of a Vatican postage stamp, the proceeds of which would go to support a home and clinic for children with AIDS in Kenya.[29]

Poverty and gender discrimination play key roles in the worldwide transmission of AIDS. Most of those infected with HIV live in developing countries, where poverty may discourage people from becoming educated about the causes of AIDS, from having access to preventive measures, and from seeking testing and treatment. Poverty also drives people to adopt risky "survival strategies," such as prostitution or the acceptance of food or school fees in return for a sexual relationship. Women, more frequently than not, lack self-determination in sexual relationships, even within marriage. Women often do not have the ability to refuse sex with their husbands, demand fidelity or AIDS testing from their husbands, or insist that an infected spouse use a condom. UN officials say young African women are three times as likely as young men to become infected with HIV. Worldwide, 48 percent of those with HIV are women, an increase of nearly a third in twenty years.[30] In Africa, women have been reported to account for 67 percent of those infected.[31] But gender imbalance in vulnerability to AIDS is certainly not limited to Africa.

What might be called a "practical theological bioethics" venture to empower women against AIDS has taken shape under the leadership of Sisters of Mercy Margaret Farley and Eileen Hogan. Farley, a feminist theologian, bioethicist, and Yale University faculty member, sought funding from USAID to begin a women's project at Yale Divinity School that became the springboard for a series of conferences in Africa.[32] Known as the All Africa Conference: Sister-to-Sister, the series is supported by international conferences of women's religious communities, in partnership with such communities in Africa. It aims to provide an opportunity for African women to come together, identify the problems they face, share experiences and strategies, and devise solutions that meet their local situations effectively. Women at Yale Divinity School have communicated with colleagues at the American Academy of Religion, the Society of Biblical Literature, and universities in the United States. They hope to inspire similar efforts and networks in Asia, Latin America, and North America. Many other "global to local" efforts to attack AIDS by changing practices and structures in the context of ordinary life have been mounted by international Catholic agencies such as Catholic Relief Services, the African Jesuit AIDS Network, Caritas International, and Symposium of Episcopal Conferences of Africa and Madagascar (SECAM). According to a Vatican representative who addressed the United Nations in 2001, 12 percent of those providing care to HIV/AIDS patients worldwide are agencies of the Catholic Church, and 13 percent are Catholic nongovernmental organizations. The Catholic Church thus provides 25 percent of the total care given to HIV/AIDS victims.[33]

Conclusion

Relationality is a basic dimension of being human, of which response is the moral heart and responsibility is the moral call. This anthropological perspective makes Catholic Christian theological bioethics a version of *social* ethics, on every issue and in every context. This is clear from biblical sources, Catholic social tradition, and the history and growing international vision of Catholic health care itself. But it is not enough for theological bioethics to *talk* about responsible relationality, or to defend it from a theoretical perspective. The wager of the Catholic common good tradition, and hence of Catholic theological bioethics, is that their grounding anthropology can be validated in practice. Authentic theological bioethics already sponsors new patterns of action, and of public social engagement, that transform relationships to enhance the common good.

NOTES

1. Catholic Health Association, *Harnessing the Promise of Genomics: Resources for Catholic Health Ministry*, Facilitator's Resource Manual (St. Louis: Catholic Health Association, 2004), 61.

2. H. Richard Niebuhr, *The Responsible Self: An Essay in Christian Moral Philosophy* (New York: Harper and Row, 1963), 65.

3. Ibid., 61–65.

4. Douglas John Hall, *Imaging God: Dominion as Stewardship* (Grand Rapids, MI: Wm. B. Eerdmans, 1986; New York: Friendship, 1986), 115.

5. Ibid., 116.

6. See, for example, Claus Westermann, *Creation*, trans. John J. Scullion (Philadelphia: Fortress Press, 1974), and *Genesis*, trans. David E. Green (Edinburgh: T&T Clark, 1995; originally published by Eerdmans, 1987). On the original meaning of "image" as a representative of an authoritative figure, such as a king, see Edward M. Curtis, "Image of God (OT)," *Anchor Bible Dictionary III*, ed. David Noel Freedman (New York: Doubleday, 1992), 390. This meaning also connotes social relationships as the arena in which the king's authority is represented and fulfilled.

7. Hall, *Imaging God*, 113.

8. See Mary Catherine Hilkert, "Imago Dei: Does the Symbol Have a Future?" (Santa Clara Lecture 8/3, Santa Clara University, Santa Clara, CA, April 14, 2002). Premodern generations of Christians read the Genesis creation stories in light of hierarchical assumptions about human relationships and the relationship of humanity to the natural world. For example, Thomas Aquinas believed that "man" in his natural, created state would have exercised a legitimate "mastership" over subordinate human beings, including women, and over animals, plants, and inanimate creatures. *Summa Theologiae*, I. Q. 96. art. 4. He believed this necessary for the common good. Moreover, humans in earlier eras were even more frequently than now at the mercy of the natural universe for their survival, a theme evident in Martin Luther's *Commentary in Genesis*. Luther laments the fact that working the land for a living is now done with great danger and difficulty, whereas in Eden this work would have been delightful. Luther, *Commentary on Genesis*, in *Luther's Works*, vol. 1, ed. Jaroslav Pelikan (Saint Louis, MO: Concordia Publishing House, 1955), 101–3. The biblical theme of human governance over the natural world, combined with the need of most humans historically to fend off threatening

natural forces, has exacerbated the sinful human tendency to deal with other creatures in a mode of aggressive dominance.

9. John Paul II, *Centesimus Annus,* no. 11, in *Catholic Social Thought: The Documentary Heritage,* ed. David J. O'Brien and Thomas A. Shannon (Maryknoll, NY: Orbis, 1998), 447.

10. Catherine Mowry LaCugna, "God in Communion with Us," in *Freeing Theology: The Essentials of Theology in Feminist Perspective,* ed. Catherine Mowry LaCugna (New York: HarperCollins, 1993), 106.

11. Ibid., 106.

12. This and the other social encyclicals may be found in David J. O'Brien and Thomas A. Shannon, eds., *Catholic Social Thought: The Documentary Heritage* (Maryknoll, NY: Orbis, 1998).

13. Second Vatican Council, *Gaudium et spes,* no. 26, in *Catholic Social Thought,* ed. O'Brien and Shannon.

14. Ibid.

15. For example, see John XXIII, *Pacem in terris,* nos. 132–39, in *Catholic Social Thought,* ed. O'Brien and Shannon, on the "universal common good."

16. See Paul VI, *Populorum progressio,* nos. 44 and 48, in *Catholic Social Teaching,* ed. O'Brien and Shannon, 250, 251.

17. John Paul II, *Sollicitudo rei socialis,* no. 38, in *Catholic Social Teaching,* ed. O'Brien and Shannon, 421.

18. See *Quadragesimo anno,* no. 70, *Mater et magistra,* no. 53, and *Pacem in terris,* no. 140, in *Catholic Social Teaching,* ed. O'Brien and Shannon.

19. *Pacem in terris,* no. 140.

20. *Sollicitudo rei socialis,* no. 39, p. 422.

21. U.S. Bishops, "Resolution on Health Care Reform," *Origins* 23, no. 7 (1993): 99, all from section 1A.

22. U.S. Census Bureau, *Income, Poverty, and Health Insurance Coverage in the United States: 2003,* August 26, 2004, available at www.census.gov/prod/2004pubs/p60-226.pdf (accessed November 21, 2005).

23. John Paul II, Tanzania, 1990, as cited in "Live and Let Live," the statement of CAFOD (Catholic Agency for Overseas Development, of Caritas International), for the World AIDS Campaign 2003–4, www.cafod.org.uk/policy_and_analysis/policy_papers/hivaids/live_and_let_live (accessed November 21, 2005).

24. Archbishop Javier Lozano Barragan, "Holy See Delegation's Address to the UN General Assembly on HIV/AIDS," June 27, 2001, www.cafod.org/uk/resources/worship/church_statements/church_s_address (accessed November 21, 2005).

25. For a discussion of participatory democracy in relation to theological bioethics, see Lisa Sowle Cahill, "Bioethics, Theology and Social Change," *Journal of Religious Ethics* 31 (2003): 3384–86.

26. Catholic Health Association, *Advocacy Agenda: 2003 and 2004* (St. Louis, MO: Catholic Health Association, 2002); for further information, see www.chausa.org.

27. Catholic Health Association, *Continuing the Commitment: A Pathway to Health Care Reform* (St. Louis, MO: Catholic Health Association, 2000). Available at www.chausa.org/PUBLICPO/PUBLICPO/asp (accessed July 30, 2004).

28. See Summary Report, "Catholic Ministries as Catalysts for Healthier Communities," available at www.chausa.org/SAB/HEALTHIER_COMMUNITIES_ASP (accessed August 2, 2004); and CHA Staff, "Collaboration the Key to Providing Care for the Uninsured," www.chausa.org/03ASSEMB/2003INSIDEM8.ASP (accessed August 24, 2004).

29. BBC News, "Vatican Condemns AIDS Drug Firms," January 29, 2004, httpc://news.bbc.co.uk/1/hi/world/europe/3442217.stm (accessed November 21, 2005). The orphanage, Nyumbani, is run by Angelo D'Agostino, S.J., an indefatigable advocate for AIDS victims and for the low-cost availability of AIDS drugs in the developing world. See also D'Agostino featured in "News Briefs," *America*, February 16, 2004, 5.

30. Michael Wines, "Women in Lesotho Become Easy Prey for H.I.V.," *New York Times*, July 30, 2004, A1.

31. Gillian Patterson, "Braving Rows and Saving Lives," *The Tablet*, July 24, 2004, 8.

32. Margaret A. Farley, "Partnership in Hope: Gender, Faith, and Responses to HIV/AIDS in Africa," *Journal of Feminist Studies in Religion* 20, no. 1 (2004): 133–48.

33. Barragan, "Address on HIV/AIDS."

PART

5

Theological Anthropology and Praxis

12

Health Care and a Theological Anthropology

Carol Taylor, C.S.F.N.

Each fall I pose the same question to the new group of chaplains and pastoral caregivers in our clinical pastoral education program. "What is it that your religious tradition invites you to 'reach into' to inform your ethical judgments about medical interventions?" Some Catholic chaplains quickly point to the *Ethical and Religious Directives for Catholic Health Care Services,* promulgated by the United States Conference of Catholic Bishops, indicating that it applies centuries of Catholic moral teaching to contemporary health care issues. When asked what grounds these teachings, they often reference scripture but are frequently at a loss when pressed to explain a judgment about something not explicitly addressed by scripture, such as embryonic stem cell research. Some who are better acquainted with the directives reference "the true dignity and vocation of the human person":

"In a time of new medical discoveries, rapid technological developments, and social change, what is new can either be an opportunity for genuine advancement in human culture, or it can lead to policies and actions that are *contrary to the true dignity and vocation of the human person*.[1] But many find the criterion of the "true dignity and vocation of the human person" unhelpful because it is open to wide and conflicting interpretations. Is withdrawing medical nutrition and hydration from the patient now diagnosed to be in persistent vegetative state (postcoma unresponsiveness) respectful or disrespectful of the dignity of the patient? Chaplains from other Christian traditions are often quick to indicate that persons must reach their own decisions about the licitness of particular medical interventions based on their personal understanding of how scripture and their relationship with God apply. Catholic teaching privileges conscience and urges Catholics to form a correct conscience based on the moral norms for proper health care. And yet when I meet with many Christians who take their faith seriously and want to make ethically good decisions about health, they are at a loss to describe how they calibrate their moral compass, without an explicit church teaching.

It is these experiences that made me eager to invite the reflection, writing, and dialogue that culminated in this book. Would reflection and dialogue that results in a rich theological anthropology provide practical guidance for those involved in the definition, design, implementation, financing, and evaluation of health care? Thus I will briefly address what a theological anthropology might contribute to health care—the focus of many chapters of this book. In the chapters that follow, Catholic ethicists involved in health policy (Ron Hamel) and science, specifically molecular genetics (Kevin FitzGerald), will more fully elaborate on its contributions in their respective disciplines.

Why Health Care Needs a Theological Anthropology

A rich theological anthropology provides guidance on how to (1) find meaning in the vulnerabilities that accompany birth, aging and its developmental challenges, acute and chronic illness, and dying; (2) organize and deliver health care; (3) approach all parties receiving and providing health care, especially the most vulnerable; (4) make individual health care decisions as both patients/surrogates and health care professionals; and (5) prioritize health decisions as institutions.

How to Find Meaning in the Vulnerabilities That Accompany Birth, Aging, and Its Developmental Challenges—Acute and Chronic Illness, and Dying
While many of the chapters in this book explore this theme, Toombs, Lysaught, and Zaner are eloquent in their descriptions of vulnerability, and in the interests of brevity I will simply reference their work.

How We Organize and Deliver Health Care
Bill Frist, U.S. Senate majority leader and physician, was asked immediately after the reelection of President George W. Bush how he thought health care needs would be addressed in the next four years. His response, "We will provide coverage for prescription drugs for some seniors, increase options for medical savings accounts, and so on," reflected the popular belief that health care is a commodity best regulated in the marketplace that privileges the wealthy and an appalling indifference to the needs of the growing numbers of the uninsured and the underinsured who lack access to basic health care services.[2] *A theological anthropology that boldly privileges our social nature and obligation to care for one another* would not allow Christian citizens to rest until health care reform radically restructures health care delivery and guarantees necessary services for all. Cahill's essay on bioethics, relationships, and participation in the common good capably explores this theme.

How We Approach All and Especially the Most Vulnerable
Central to a Christian theological anthropology is the conviction that *each human person is created in the image of God and redeemed by Christ* and thus we are all the same in our ontological or inherent dignity, worth, and claim for respect. This conviction does not rest peacefully side by side with the national studies in the United States demonstrating glaring disparities in health outcomes based purely on race and ethnicity, not to mention socioeconomic status or other variables such as gender, sexual orientation, lifestyle variables, body size, and so on. A Christian theological anthropology would boldly challenge all unjust relationships that objectify and demean individuals be they patients, family members, or other members of the team—professional or lay, and community and populations groups.

How Individuals, Patients/Surrogates, and Health Care Professionals Make Health Care Decisions
We have a history in the United States of medicalizing health care in a way that is inconsistent with respectful care and human flourishing. Excesses

of medicalization and inappropriate uses of technology begged for reforms in childbirth and end-of-life care that culminated respectively in the natural childbirth and hospice and palliative care movements. Slow to learn from our mistakes, we are now repeating them in the prenatal arena (are parents who refuse to do everything in their power to produce a "perfect" child—i.e., quality control measures—morally irresponsible?) and in genomic medicine.

A Christian theological anthropology *views humans as finite creatures of a loving creator, called to be cocreators of this world, and ultimately destined for the full perfection of human life—not in the here and now, but with eternal union with God.* Such a view takes seriously the fact that life is a gift, not ours to initiate or terminate, but just the same, a gift to be appreciated and stewarded carefully. This view demands humble reflection on what it means to choose freely in accord with God's plan versus the capricious maximization of individual preferences to invent some new desirable *me.* See Margaret Mohrmann's and Suzanne Holland's essays on integrity.

Furthermore, regarding end-of-life care issues, I am always struck by those who fight death on demand by retreating to a type of vitalism that basically tells God, "You cannot have this life." To the extent that we believe that there is a point at which God calls us each "home," the challenge is to discern when is this moment and then to gracefully accept the invitation and go, which would entail a graceful "letting go" by both patients and those who love them. A theological anthropology that accepts human finitude would be a serious challenge to our death-denying culture and would resist the notion that only Kevorkian-type deaths are "good deaths." Catholic hospitals continue to believe that they cannot "market" good dying—because it would be "bad for business." "People come here to be cured, not to die!" Richard Zaner's meditation on vulnerability and power in this book explores this concept in profound ways.

How Institutions and Systems Make Health Care Decisions
Health care institutions are primarily healing institutions, but they are also employers, business partners, and corporate citizens. A rich theological anthropology has the potential to influence not only the services ("product lines") a Catholic or Christian institution provides ("Should we offer prenatal genetic counseling?") but also its business decisions (socially responsible investing, honest marketing, refraining from cut-throat competition), its employee relations (just wages and benefit packages, safe working environments), and its corporate citizen responsibilities (case mix: provision of

services to most needy). A theological anthropology cognizant of salvation history reminds us that sin is a reality for both individuals and collectives, and it cautions us to be alert to the faces idolatry, greed, injustice, dishonesty, and other forms of social sin wear in the workplace and society.

Conclusion

I have always argued that those of us involved in health care need to keep our attention firmly fixed on the human consequences of our decisions and actions. That is, while scientific, clinical, economic, and legal lenses are all essential, our primary focus should be how people, and in particular, people made vulnerable by illness and other factors, will be affected by who we choose to be as we engage in healing encounters and make and implement decisions about health care design, implementation, financing, and evaluation.

NOTES

1. Emphasis mine. National Catholic Conference of Bishops/United States Catholic Conference, *Ethical and Religious Directives for Catholic Health Care Services,* 4th ed. (Washington, DC: United States Conference of Catholic Bishops, 2001). Available at www.usccb.org/bishops/directives.htm (accessed January 24, 2005).

2. W. H. Frist, "Shattuck Lecture: Health Care in the 21st Century," special article, *New England Journal of Medicine* 352, no. 2 (2005): 267–72.

CHAPTER

13

Health Policy and a Theological Anthropology

Ron Hamel

In all probability, many policymakers as well as a good number of our fellow citizens (including some bioethicists) would look askance at the juxtaposition of the terms "health policy" and "theological anthropology." Assuming they know what a theological anthropology is, some might, at best, wonder about the relevance of such a thing to the very practical concerns of policy making. How could something so theoretical and even esoteric have any bearing on shaping health policy? Others might become concerned or even fearful at the joining of the two terms. Their combination conjures up worries about the separation of church and state, the place of religion in a pluralistic society, and the often acrimonious and intransigent responses of some religious groups to current and proposed public policy.[1]

Most likely, neither policymakers nor society at large are waiting for a theological anthropology to help inform public policy on issues relating to biomedicine. The social and political climates, however, are no reason to dismiss the potential significance of a theological anthropology or attempts to articulate such an anthropology and its implications for health policy. But they should have a sobering effect, reminding us that an already difficult task is made even more difficult by skepticism, fear, or outright hostility. The task is well worth undertaking, I believe, because a theological anthropology might help to address significant lacunae in the societal ethos that currently informs our public policy relating to biomedicine.

In what follows, I address three questions: (1) Why does public policy relating to bioethics need a theological anthropology? (2) What might a theological anthropology contribute to health policy, generally and specifically? (3) What are some of the challenges that a theological anthropology faces in relation to health policy? In order to further focus this discussion, I will use as a case in point the current public policy debate over embryonic stem cell research.

Why a Theological Anthropology for Health Policy?

Appearing before the Democratic National Convention on July 27, 2004, Ron Reagan pleaded his case for a change in the current policy regarding the use of government funds for embryonic stem cell research. His comments illustrate well the major arguments advanced in support of such research. First, there is the possibility that embryonic stem cells will be able to provide cures for a wide range of diseases and medical conditions and thereby alleviate enormous pain and suffering for so many. "Millions are afflicted," said Reagan, "[a]nd every year, every day, tragedy is visited upon families across the country, around the world. Now, it may be within our power to put an end to this suffering. We need only try."[2] Second, we have an *obligation* to relieve the pain and suffering of others by whatever means we have at our disposal. Those who obstruct funding for embryonic stem cell research bear some responsibility for the future suffering and possibly the deaths of others.[3] "What excuse will we offer this young woman should we fail her now? What might we tell her children? Or the millions of others who suffer? That when given an opportunity to help, we turned away? That facing political opposition, we lost our nerve? That even though we knew better, we did nothing. . . . No, no, we owe this young woman and all those who suffer—we owe ourselves—better than that."[4]

Third, we need to pursue knowledge for its own sake and to do so in an unfettered manner. Freedom of thought, freedom of conscience, and freedom of inquiry are paramount.[5] "We are motivated by a thirst for knowledge."[6] Fourth, the destruction of embryos to obtain stem cells is justified. The pain and suffering of those in need and free scientific inquiry should outweigh any concerns for embryos.[7] "Now, there are those who would stand in the way of this remarkable future, who would deny the federal funding so crucial to basic research. They argue that interfering with the development of even the earliest stage embryo, even one that will never be implanted in a womb and will never develop into an actual fetus, is tantamount to murder. . . . Yes, these cells could theoretically have the potential, under very different circumstances, to develop into human beings—that potential is where their magic lies. But they are not, in and of themselves, human beings."[8]

What do these arguments say about the need for a theological anthropology in the debate about public funding of embryonic stem cell research particularly and about health policy generally? Most often, public policy discussions, because they tend to be so pragmatic, reflect a somewhat limited perspective or vision. The discussions are fairly narrowly defined and immediately focused. Hence they lack breadth and depth. There is more at stake, for example, than the formulation of the policy itself. Such policy choices also have a bearing on how it is we conceive what it means to be human and on what kind of individuals and society we become. "In biomedicine," says theologian Hubert Doucet, "our human identity is at stake. So the basic bioethical question is: 'What humanity do we want to become?'"[9] Or, in the words of Hugh Heclo, "Technological advances have brought our nation to the point where profoundly important public choices are becoming inescapable. . . . [T]echnological society . . . demands public policy choices with ever more far reaching consequences for the meaning of human life . . . policy choices drenched in religious and cultural implications as to what humankind is and how we should live."[10] Both authors point to the fact that embedded in debates about public policy with regard to biomedicine are questions of meaning that more often than not are not even recognized or, if recognized, are not engaged. Advances in biomedicine, because they touch on such fundamental dimensions of human life and human life lived together, inevitably raise questions of meaning. Neglecting questions of meaning—questions about what it means to be human, what it means to live in society, what constitutes human life, how we might understand illness and disability, human finitude, suffering and death, progress, the pursuit of knowledge, the place of science in human life and society—can only have adverse consequences for us as individuals and as a society in the long run.

Insight into these questions of meaning cannot come from science. Nor are they likely to come from a culture that has such a thin understanding of the human as does ours. Theology and, more specifically, theological anthropology can provide such insights, can help fill the need created by the unrelenting advance of technology. Again, to quote Heclo: "There is no escaping a future where religious faith intertwines with the politics of policymaking."[11] So what is it that a theological anthropology might contribute to public policy in biomedicine?

Theological Anthropology and Health Policy: Potential Contributions

I suggest six ways in which a fulsome theological anthropology might contribute directly and indirectly to public policy in biomedicine. First, and rather obviously, it can provide a far richer understanding of what it means to be human than what is currently operative in American society and in public policy formation. In the words of James Walter, "Theology can continue to contribute to bioethics issues [and, I would add, to public policy] by focusing not merely on procedures but primarily on the substantive meaning of the nature of persons."[12] An understanding of the human person that has breadth and depth—that goes beyond an emphasis on the individual, on autonomy, and on individual rights—could lead to public policy that will better contribute to the flourishing of individuals and society.

In the embryonic stem cell debate, the moral status of the embryo is surely a primary consideration. What is the nature of a human embryo, and what do we owe it?[13] But this is not the only anthropological consideration. A theological anthropology would also want to underscore our social nature and the duties we have toward and responsibilities we have for one another, including nascent human life and those who suffer from disease and disability. This includes what we become as individuals and as a society in and through the choices we make. What will be the impact on us and on those who come after us if we accept the destruction of nascent human life? What will be the impact on us if we acquiesce to using nascent human life for *our* purposes? This theological anthropology would want to consider what we owe one another in our various social interactions, that is, what justice requires of us. Who will benefit from the cures, if any, developed from embryonic stem cells? Who will have access to such treatments?[14] Will we ensure fair access and equitable distribution?

Such an anthropology would likely consider the fact that human beings are finite, that limitations of various kinds—illness, disability, and death among them—are an ultimately inescapable part of our life experience. Human beings are in the odd situation of being essentially limited while always striving to transcend limitation. A theological anthropology would also likely consider human sinfulness, the fact that so often we pursue and choose to do what is contrary to respect for human dignity and human flourishing. It would underscore the fact that often we pursue the wrong goals, or the right goals for the wrong reasons or in the wrong ways. Power, greed, and hubris are powerful forces that can lead us off the mark.

A second and very much related contribution is that a broader and deeper understanding of what it means to be human can in turn lead to an expansion of the considerations that enter into discussions of public policy in biomedicine. Our public policy discussions usually become narrowly construed focusing on, for example, rights individualistically understood, or procedures to ensure noninterference, or the pragmatic results and benefits of particular technologies. The embryonic stem cell debate is focused on the moral status of the embryo, the hoped-for benefits of the research, a presumed obligation to pursue this research for the benefit of others, and an unfettered pursuit of knowledge. These are undoubtedly all critical considerations. But there are more, as was suggested earlier, in identifying some aspects of a theological anthropology and some of their implications for embryonic stem cell research. By broadening our considerations, by paying attention to more of what is at stake, one hopes for a policy that has taken account of the complexities of these situations and hence becomes a more fitting response for the good of society.

Third, a fulsome theological anthropology of necessity raises questions of meaning. In public policy discussions, questions of meaning are there invariably, but, as already noted, they are most often not recognized or, if recognized, are not engaged. A culture marked by classical liberalism and a hypersensitivity toward pluralism is not inclined to take on questions of meaning. But this is to the detriment of public policy and society. It results in thin discussions, inadequate readings of what is going on and of what is at stake, and usually, a public policy that reflects this. In the embryonic stem cell debate, the meaning questions go beyond the moral status of the embryo. They encompass other things such as how we understand illness, disability and death, our finitude, how we deal with limitation as well as the drive to overcome it, our obligations to others and to future generations to seek and provide cures for disease and disability, the common good, scientific progress, and the pursuit of knowledge. Surely policymakers, in their deliberations, will not spend much if any time pondering such questions. However, it is quite possible that some sectors of society would, and that this in turn could affect the nature of deliberations and the shape of policy proposals.

Fourth, a theological anthropology could serve a prophetic function with regard to public policy in biomedicine. It could remind society of critical dimensions that are not being considered; challenge beliefs and values that ultimately do not contribute to human flourishing; point to the consequences for individuals and society of certain values, convictions, and choices; and call society to be and seek to become more. A theological anthropology, for example, could invite society to reflect on its attitude toward nascent human life and its obligations toward that life and all the vulnerable in our midst. It might call into question a mentality and a practice that is willing to sacrifice the most vulnerable for the benefit of many and, concomitantly, the use of a utilitarian calculus in the development of public policy. It might call for examination of the assumption that we *must* pursue every avenue available to us in the great desire to relieve pain and suffering. In its prophetic role, a theological anthropology might challenge the technological imperative and might raise up for consideration the variety of motives behind the drive to make use of embryonic stem cells, including profit, prestige, and power. It might hold up for reflection and debate the possible impact of our choices about this issue on our very humanity and upon the kind of society we become.

Fifth, a theological anthropology has the potential for transforming the community of believers, all of whom are citizens and some of whom are policymakers. All of us operate out of a particular worldview, a particular way of seeing and interpreting reality. That worldview affects what is seen and not seen, what is valued and not valued, what is valued more and what is valued less. All of us bring these values, beliefs, dispositions, intentions, motives, and sentiments to our deliberations and our judgments. One of the primary indirect contributions of a theological anthropology to health policy is to influence the worldview of members of the faith community. Surely not all would incorporate dimensions of a theological anthropology into their worldview. They might prefer dimensions of other theological anthropologies or even other worldviews. This contribution of a theological anthropology to public policy in biomedicine, however, hinges on at least two things. One is education or formation, the gradual shaping of the character of individual believers. How is this done and done deliberately, consistently and successfully? The other is dialogue, communities of believers functioning also as communities of moral discourse, exploring moral issues in light of their faith and their theological understanding of what it means to be human. If these two things can occur successfully, it is more likely that a theological anthropology will have some effect on the formulation of public policy.

Sixth, and finally, a theological anthropology can help shape Catholic (and perhaps even Catholic-Christian) policy proposals. The United States Conference of Catholic Bishops, state Catholic conferences, Catholic Charities, the Catholic Health Association, and other Catholic organizations are almost constantly either responding to policy proposals at the federal and state levels or initiating or cosponsoring such proposals. It is inconceivable that these activities would not be grounded in a Catholic-Christian worldview and a Catholic-Christian understanding of the human person. A theological anthropology could shore up this grounding and could also have the deepening and broadening effect discussed earlier.[15] The Catholic community, in its public policy deliberations, is not beyond narrow considerations.

Theological Anthropology and Health Policy: Challenges

The relationship of a theological anthropology to public policy in biomedicine is not without its difficulties. Many could undoubtedly be noted. I call attention to four. The first has to do with language and communication. We are a society of Catholics and other-than-Catholics, of believers and unbelievers. If the insights of a theological anthropology are to have any effect on the development and formulation of public policy, those insights cannot be expressed in esoteric language, that is, in language that is specifically tied to the Catholic faith community or even the Christian tradition. The insights of our theological tradition and of a theological anthropology must be communicated with all their power in a manner that is comprehensible to the general public without diluting the richness of our theological symbol.[16]

Another challenge is the plurality of theological anthropologies, even within the Catholic community. There is not just one theological anthropology. In fact, many exist. While there may be some strong commonalities among them, there are also serious differences. In some cases, those differences can be mutually enriching. In other cases, however, the differences are not complementary. They are more or less contradictory. How will those differences be negotiated? Which interpretations of what it means to be human will prevail? An obvious case in point is the plurality of views about the moral status of the human embryo, even within the Catholic community. One could also point to differences in understanding what it means to be made in the *imago dei* and the implications of those understandings for interpreting the human-creation relationship.

The third challenge concerns the move from a theological anthropology to public policy. The notions of human dignity, respect for human life, solidarity, justice, human finitude, and the like do not automatically translate into specific policy proposals, even assuming there is clarity about the concepts themselves and their implications. In the words of Kenneth and Michael Himes, "Theology must be mediated by social ethics before it makes specific judgments about action. It is simplistic politically and fundamentalistic theologically to ignore the mediating role of social ethics. While the God of the Hebrew and Christian scriptures has concern for the poor, the weak and the exile, that claim is hardly sufficient in itself for determining the details of taxation, welfare reform, regulation of private property or other societal policies."[17] It is unlikely that social ethics alone can serve that mediating role in the domain of bioethics. But it would seem to be the case that social ethics constitutes a part of those mediating structures.

A final challenge in bringing a theological anthropology to bear on public policy regarding biomedicine is *how* that will be accomplished. In addition to mediating principles, there would also seem to be a need for other mediating entities and processes—individuals who have been shaped by a worldview that is constituted in part by a theological anthropology whether explicitly or implicitly, communities of moral discourse, civil and reasoned dialogues with those outside the community of faith, various forms of education, policy proposals, and advocacy, among them. The great danger, of course, is that theology becomes ideology, that truth is perceived to exist on one side only, that persuasion is replaced by assertions and dialogue by monologue, shouting, and intolerance, and that one position must always win out in an all or nothing manner. Such developments would severely undermine the critical, positive contributions of a theological anthropology to public policy in biomedicine. They could even have the effect of once again marginalizing the role of religion and theology in the public square.

Conclusion

Writing about public policy relating to stem cell research, Margaret McLean says,

White-knuckled, we are crossing medical frontiers at break neck speed. Stem cell technology holds the promise not only of increasing human health and life spans but also of changing power structures and fundamental notions of personhood, moral status, and mortality. It is important that we do not prematurely or unwittingly slam the door on scientific advances that can relieve human suffering and restore health. At the same time, it is imperative that, in this biotechnologic age, we expand our moral imaginations to account for and be accountable to marginalized persons and concern ourselves with the shaping of a just future.[18]

The need to expand our moral imaginations is true with respect to not only embryonic stem cell research but also a host of other biomedical technologies and issues relating to health care. Much is clearly at stake. The public policy choices we make today will define us as a society and will undoubtedly affect future generations in profound ways. A theological anthropology for bioethics can help to expand our moral imaginations so that we will not one day regret the policy choices we make today. They will be choices that truly respect human dignity and contribute to human flourishing.

NOTES

1. For various discussions of the relationship of religion and public policy in the United States, see Hugh Heclo and Wilfred M. McClay, eds., *Religion Returns to the Public Square: Faith and Policy in America* (Washington, DC: Woodrow Wilson Center Press, 2003). See also Ronald F. Thiemann, *Religion in Public Life: A Dilemma for Democracy* (Washington, DC: Georgetown University Press, 1996).

2. Ron Reagan, "Ron Reagan's Remarks at the Democratic Convention," www.usatoday.com/news/politicselections/nation/president/2004-07-29-reagan-speech-text_x.htm (accessed January 19, 2006).

3. President's Council on Bioethics, *Monitoring Stem Cell Research* (Washington, DC: U.S. Government Printing Office, 2004), 58, 59.

4. Reagan, "Remarks at the Democratic Convention."

5. President's Council, *Monitoring Stem Cell Research,* 61.

6. Reagan, "Remarks at the Democratic Convention."

7. President's Council, *Monitoring Stem Cell Research,* 58, 62–63.

8. Reagan, "Remarks at the Democratic Convention." A very similar rationale to the preceding is offered in a June 22, 2004, letter to President Bush from the International Society for Stem Cell Research as well as in an April 28, 2004, letter to the president from 206 members of the House of Representatives and an identical June 4, 2004, letter from fifty-eight members of the Senate.

9. Hubert Doucet, "How Theology Could Contribute to the Redemption of Bioethics from an Individualist Approach to an Anthropological Sensitivity," *The Catholic Theological Society of America Proceedings* 53 (1998): 61.

10. Hugh Heclo, "An Introduction to Religion and Public Policy," in *Religion Returns to the Public Square: Faith and Policy in America*, ed. Hugh Heclo and Wilfred M. McClay (Washington, DC: Woodrow Wilson Center Press, 2003), 22, 23.

11. Ibid., 23.

12. James Walter, "A Response to Hubert Doucet," *The Catholic Theological Society of America Proceedings* 53 (1998): 70.

13. There is an extensive literature that deals with this topic. See, for example, Lisa Sowle Cahill, "The Embryo and the Fetus: New Moral Contexts," *Theological Studies* 54 (March 1993): 124–42; Margaret Farley, "Roman Catholic Views on Research Involving Human Embryonic Stem Cells," in *The Human Embryonic Stem Cell Debate: Science, Ethics, and Public Policy*, ed. Suzanne Holland, Karen Lebacqz, and Lauri Zoloth (Cambridge, MA: MIT Press, 2001), 113–18; John Collins Harvey, "Distinctly Human: The When, Where and Why of Life's Beginnings," *Commonweal* 129, no. 3 (2002): 11–13; Paul Lauritzen, "Neither Person nor Property," *America* 184, no. 10 (2001): 20–23; Richard A. McCormick, "Who or What Is the Preembryo?" in *Corrective Vision* (Kansas City, MO: Sheed & Ward, 1994): 176–88; Michael Panicola, "Three Views of the Preimplantation Embryo," *National Catholic Bioethics Quarterly* 2, no. 1 (2002): 69–97; Jean Porter, "Is the Embryo a Person?" *Commonweal* 129, no. 3 (2002): 8–10; Carol Tauer, "The Tradition of Probabilism and the Moral Status of the Early Embryo," *Theological Studies* 45 (1984): 3–33.

14. See, for example, Lisa Sowle Cahill, "The New Biotech World Order," *Hastings Center Report* 29, no. 2 (1999): 45–48; Ronald P. Hamel et al., "A Catholic Vision toward Genomic Advances" (St. Louis, MO: Catholic Health Association, 2004), 12; Margaret R. McClean, "Stem Cells: Shaping the Future in Public Policy," in *The Human Embryonic Stem Cell Debate*, ed. Holland, Lebacqz, and Zoloth, 202–4.

15. See John A. Coleman, "American Catholicism, Catholic Charities USA, and Welfare Reform," in *Religion Returns to the Public Square: Faith and Policy in America*, ed. Heclo and McClay, 229–67.

16. See Lisa Sowle Cahill, "Can Theology Have a Role in 'Public' Bioethical Discourse?" *Hastings Center Report*, special supplement, 20, no. 4 (1990): 10–14; Bryan Hehir, "Policy Arguments in a Public Church: Social Ethics and Bioethics," *Journal of Medicine and Philosophy* 17, no. 3 (1992): 347–64; Michael J. Himes and Kenneth R. Himes, "The Public Church and Public Theology," *Fullness of Faith: The Public Significance of Theology* (Mahwah, NJ: Paulist Press, 1993), 1–27.

17. Himes and Himes, "Public Church," 22.

18. McClean, "Stem Cells," 205.

CHAPTER

14

Science and a Theological Anthropology

Kevin T. FitzGerald, S.J.

Like scientific investigation, theological-anthropological reflection is an ongoing activity—one that must be engaged in active reflection upon and interaction with the findings of the natural sciences. Certainly, our understanding of human anatomy and physiology, human development, biochemistry, genetics, psychology—in short, every aspect of human nature that has been examined and investigated by the natural sciences—has changed radically over the course of history, particularly over the past several decades. Scientific investigation and biotechnical innovation will undoubtedly bring with them new challenges to our conceptions of human nature, human flourishing, and theological anthropology. Recently, the president's council on bioethics (2003) and the National Science Foundation et al. (2004) have brought to our attention the variety of ways in which biotechnology may come to bear on human life in the near future and thereby the variety of questions that will be raised concerning whether, or how, human life may be enhanced by biotechnology. We need to discern what science is revealing about our nature and how this revelation might combine with revelation (along with other forms of knowledge) to give us a richer and deeper understanding of how humans thrive and whether, how, or to what extent we are called to go "beyond therapy" or "beyond" human nature.

Can We Go Beyond Human Nature?

Answering this question completely would require addressing it on many different levels, including the debated issues of whether or not there is such a thing as human nature, and whether consideration of human nature should be included in serious reflection about the uses of technology.[1] For the sake of brevity, it can be observed that there have been many responses to these issues from a variety of perspectives, all of which argue for the inclusion of some concept of human nature in this discussion.[2] Then, regardless of which concept of human nature one chooses to employ, one still has to determine what exactly technology can do to human beings on a biological level in order to discuss whether or not any of it should be pursued.

Fundamentally, one can conclude from the current state of science and technology that almost any level of biological manipulation is possible. In other words, the biological substratum of human beings is open to manipulation from the level of prosthetic devices and artificial organs to the level of proteins, DNA, and molecular biology. Perhaps what is most pertinent to the focus of this chapter is the fact that this manipulation is not limited to interchanging human parts, though this is already clear in the case of prosthetic devices. However, our relative comfort with and support for prostheses as they are used today may not easily translate to the devices and biological interventions of the future. Two examples may help to clarify this point.

Heart valves taken from pigs or cows are currently in use to replace damaged human heart valves. This therapeutic intervention currently receives broad support. Because efforts are underway to genetically engineer pigs so that their organs would be less likely to be rejected when transplanted into human beings, one can conclude that there will be similar support for transplanting pig hearts into humans in order to save the lives of people who would otherwise die. If the pigs can provide hearts, though, what would prevent the use of other organs and tissues in humans as needed? Would there be a different reaction to the use of pig neural tissue in the brains of people with neurodegenerative diseases? If all these interventions are to be considered desirable, should we use the genetically engineered pig stem cells to replace and repair damaged tissue, if enough human stem cells are not available—or even human stem cells or tissues grown in pigs, or other mammals, to provide even more compatible tissue? Of course, for the sake of efficiency, one would want a pig with a high percentage of human cells in whatever tissues might be needed. Hence, following this line of reasoning, the optimal therapeutic answer would be a chimeric pig/human, or perhaps a chimp/human. Mammalian chimeras have already been created, such as goat/sheep "geeps," which are created by fusing a goat embryo with a sheep embryo. One can also get chimeric animals with a relatively small percentage of cells from one animal by placing stem cells from one animal into the embryo or fetus of another animal. Chimeras of this type have been made with human stem cells being placed into the embryos or fetuses of other mammals including mice, sheep, and pigs. While providing interesting research models and potentially useful sources of transplantable human tissue, these animals also raise challenging issues regarding common sense notions of the separation of species and the special status of human beings.

These blurred lines among mammalian species are not the only lines being manipulated by advances in cellular biology. Embryonic stem cell research is also providing new insights and manipulations across gender lines. Using mouse embryonic stem cells, researchers[3] have been able to obtain cells that look and function like sperm and eggs. Interestingly, both sperm and eggs can be obtained from the same embryonic stem cell line. This result indicates that an embryonic stem cell line from a male could supply eggs for fertilization, and a female embryonic stem cell line could supply sperm—or each embryonic stem cell line could supply both eggs and sperm. Considering the current emphasis in the infertility industry for parents to have genetically related children, might this emphasis on genetic relatedness combined with this technological manipulation of gametes lead to a blurring of the traditional concepts or roles of father and mother, as either or each could provide sperm or egg? Of course, one could argue that these traditional roles are already undergoing change in our society. In that case, this type of technological manipulation could be seen as increasing the rate of that change or as precipitating a more broad and deep discussion of what these roles should be and why.

What Is Beyond?

The two examples presented earlier are but discrete points along a rapidly expanding spectrum of possible biological manipulations that can be done to human beings. This spectrum also includes manipulations of everything from genetic material to artificial organs and can involve interchange among individuals and species. Such biological plasticity leads some to propose a desire for or right to what Nick Bostrom calls "morphological freedom." "From this perspective, altering our bodies, even in substantive and radical ways, is an increasingly effective way for people to become better than well."[4] However, one does not need to invoke cutting-edge technologies to encounter significant difficulties with this idea. Again, an example may help to clarify this point.

Though there has been a sizeable increase in the number and type of cosmetic surgery procedures performed in the United States and internationally (perhaps as an early impetus in some societies toward a type of morphological freedom), some surgical interventions do raise societal concerns even when only consenting adults are involved. Dr. Robert Smith,[5] a surgeon in Scotland, became embroiled in a medical controversy when it was revealed, in January 2000, that he had removed parts of healthy limbs from two patients (one in 1997, and one in 1999). Both patients had been diagnosed as suffering from Body Dysmorphic Disorder—a psychological pathology that involves a person's strong desire to have certain parts of one's body removed even though they are healthy and normal.

Dr. Smith defended his decision (which was supported by the hospital's ethics committee) by stating that each patient had been unsuccessfully treated by more conventional means and consequently were in danger of harming themselves. He could then claim that he was insuring them a lesser harm by sparing them the drastic measure of cutting off the limbs themselves, while giving them the benefit of presumably ending their suffering. His argument is obviously grounded in a particular evaluation of harms and benefits—a particular evaluation that was not shared with all others in the medical profession, as evidenced by the controversy it created.

This case highlights the difficulties that are already encountered in medicine when even relatively common technologies (i.e., surgery) are applied to situations where the harms and benefits are not clear. Did Dr. Smith really help these patients as he claimed, or did he actually harm them more by reinforcing their psychological pathologies and damaging otherwise healthy limbs? How much more will current scientific information and the coming technological interventions exacerbate these difficulties, especially with a growing diversity of opinion and argument even within the medical profession itself?

Another, perhaps more subtle, example of this difficulty can be seen in two of the targets suggested by those who would biologically go beyond our current human condition. Intelligence and care or affection for others are often cited by proponents of improving the human species as two primary targets for such improvement.[6] However, it may not be as simple to focus on these targets as technological improvement proponents appear to assume.

For instance, there are many different kinds of intelligence.[7] However, not all are readily quantifiable for scientific purposes, and not all are addressed best through the use of a scientific methodology.[8] In addition, many particularly intelligent and talented people also exhibit severe antisocial behaviors, which seem to be biologically connected to that type and level of intellectual ability.[9] In fact, severe levels of antisocial behavior may be crucial in the more extreme development of certain types of genius. Add to these findings about intelligence the experience of unconditional love that many who have worked with Down's syndrome children and adults have had, and one can easily question any claims that both intelligence and compassion will be biologically identified and enhanced in anyone by any technological means. In spite of technological utopian claims for precisely and incrementally going beyond human nature, much current scientific research is demonstrating that the characteristics most often cited as being quintessentially human, such as intelligence and compassion, have complex and interrelated biological foundations. In fact, scientific research has shown that even simple genetic diseases, such as sickle-cell anemia and cystic fibrosis, can have beneficial aspects to them, such as resistance to malaria and bubonic plague respectively. Hence curing the disease can also cause harm by increasing susceptibility to another disease.

In all, as much as science and technology are revealing a heretofore unimagined malleability in the human biological constitution, they are also revealing even more complexity and interrelatedness than had previously been suspected. The powerful, reductionistic methodology of science is actually uncovering, especially, the integrated wholeness of human beings. Therefore, any claims to going beyond human nature in some positive sense will have to address and evaluate the effects any changes will have on this integrated wholeness.

Conclusion

Contrary to what has often been stated by proponents of human embryonic stem cell research and human cloning, when they lament that religion, ethics, and politics are getting in the way of science, this is not a scientific question. The reductionistic methodologies of science, though indeed powerful, cannot grasp the richness and integration of the human condition. For this richness to be grasped, the revelations of science need to be integrated with the insights of revelation, as well as all the other ways we come to know ourselves and our condition. Thus scientists must sit down with theologians, philosophers, and even nurses and physicians, and engage in constructive dialogue. Otherwise, those who would take us beyond our human nature may, instead, drag us beneath it.

NOTES

1. See D. Cockburn, ed., *Human Beings* (New York: Cambridge University Press, 1991).

2. Examples of these different approaches include analytic philosophers such as D. Cockburn, *Other Human Beings* (New York: St. Martin's, 1990), and William Alston, "Perceiving God," *The Journal of Philosophy* 83, no. 11 (1986): 655–65, who interpret this rejection of the concept of human nature to be the result of a misguided epistemology and a false competition between physical science explanations and everyday explanations of human relationships. Feminists, such as Annette Baier, "Extending the Limits of Moral Theory," *The Journal of Philosophy* 83, no. 10 (1986): 538–45, emphasize the need to be more inclusive of concepts of human nature in our moral theories. Sociohistorical philosophers (C. Taylor, *Sources of Self* [Cambridge, MA: Harvard University Press, 1989]) and those focusing on praxis (R. Bernstein, *Beyond Objectivism and Relativism* [Philadelphia: University of Pennsylvania Press, 1988]) argue for moral discourse to expand and not rigidly to limit its scope so that it can be more relevant in addressing contemporary ethical concerns such as biotechnology.

3. M. A. Surani, "Stem Cells: How to Make Eggs and Sperm," *Nature* 427 (2004): 106–7.

4. N. Bostrom, "Human Enhancement: Answering the Why Question," available at www.transhumanism.org/tv/2004/BostromonWhy.ppt (accessed January 24, 2005).

5. British Broadcasting Company (BBC) News, "Surgeon Defends Amputations," available at http://news.bbc.co.uk/2/hi/uk_news/scotland/625680.stm (accessed January 29, 2005).

6. In addition to the Transhumanists, earlier works also mentioned these goals. For example, see J. Glover, *What Sort of People Should There Be?* (New York, Penguin, 1984); D. Suzuki and P. Knudtsen, *Genethics* (Cambridge, MA: Harvard University Press, 1989); L. M. Silver, *Remaking Eden* (New York: Perennial/Avon, 1997); and L. Walters, J. G. Palmer, and N. C. Johnson, *The Ethics of Human Gene Therapy* (New York: Oxford University Press, 1996).

7. H. Gardner, *Multiple Intelligences* (New York: Basic Books, 1993).

8. Cf. H. J. Eysenck, *Intelligence: A New Look* (New Brunswick: Transaction, 1998).

9. F. Post, "Creativity and Psychopathology," *British Journal of Psychiatry* 165 (1994): 27–34.

Toward a Richer Bioethics: A Conclusion

Edmund D. Pellegrino

> We have sought as best we can to clarify, promote and defend "being human." Where might we seek help in thinking about "life lived humanly."
> —President's Council on Bioethics, *Being Human*

In these words, President Bush's council on bioethics expressed its need for a "richer bioethics" with which to confront the challenges to our humanity inherent in the human use of contemporary biotechnology.[1] The council thus reminded itself, and all of us, of the pertinence for bioethics of what Ernst Cassirer rightly called "the Archimedean point, the fixed and immovable center of all thought."[2] By this he meant the question of man's self-knowledge, the anthropological question "What is man?"

This is the question set aside by previous committees, commissions, and reports. Yet it is the foundation stone on which the theory and content of any system of bioethics is ultimately set. It is the question that can no longer be taken for granted. In the end, the way we answer this question frames the wide range of different norms, principles, values, or intuitions that characterize today's bioethical discourse.

If we do not know who and what it means to be human, how can we judge whether the prodigious powers of biomedical science threaten or enhance our humanity? Where else can we find the template with which to measure our attempts to benefit humankind?

Since antiquity, the best minds of every era have addressed the question of man. Among modern philosophers, Max Scheler is perhaps the most acute in his interest and observation of our problem today. We have a plethora of theories of man; it is the reconciliation of the many sources of information that is so crucial today. "We have a scientific, philosophical and a theological anthropology which know nothing of each other. . . . The ever growing multiplicity of the sciences studying man has much more confused and obscured than elucidated our concept of man."[3] The president's council clearly has many ways to which it may turn. The question is how to do justice to sources that are multiple, diverse, and often strongly in opposition to each other.

Whether the president's council, or any other body, can surmount these difficulties is problematic. What is clear is that overtly, or covertly, there is an idea or image of man at the heart of most tendentious bioethical issues of the day—abortion, euthanasia, assisted suicide, end-of-life decisions, stem cell research, cloning, genomic engineering, human enhancements, and so on. The list assuredly will grow, and with it the necessity for more direct confrontation with what we mean about being human.

Today we must confront these complex issues without the traditional reliance on religion and metaphysics. The Enlightenment stripped these away and left us with autonomous reason; the idealist philosophers then turned away from external reality to mental constructs and consciousness. Under the influence of psychology and psychoanalysis, postmodernists completed the demolition by undermining the claims of reason to know external reality or moral truth. Man now face the most complex challenges in history to their humanity equipped only with their autonomous self-defined subjective humanity.[4]

These difficulties do not absolve bioethics of its neglect of the anthropological question. At the minimum, there is an obligation to try to bring the sciences dealing with man together with philosophy and theology, in an effort to find some agreed-upon set of norms to guide our private and public decision making. In bioethics, an initial attempt is being made by UNESCO's International Bioethics Committee (2005). This effort underscores the difficulties as well as the opportunities of a global effort to confront man's tenuous future in the new world of biotechnology.

Other chapters in this book confront the anthropological question tangentially, with reflections on the human phenomena of vulnerability, suffering, disease, finitude, and existential anguish. As one might expect, different images and ideas of man emerge. They reinforce the need for serious dialogue between, and among, these differing ideas when moral decisions must be made personally or politically. Dell'Oro does confront the barriers and opportunities of dialogue between bioethics and one clearly stated idea and image of man—that of Roman Catholic moral theology.[5] He offers a framework for opening a dialogue that will be mutually beneficial.

In this conclusion, I examine the nontheological anthropologies implicit or explicit in modern bioethical discourse. My aim is to provide a topography of these anthropologies, to show the way the presuppositions of each about the nature of man expresses itself in bioethics and the importance of a more open and explicit dialogue between, and among, them if the effects of biotechnology on human life are to be better understood.

A Bioethically Relevant Typology of Anthropologies

Ever since he has had the power for reflective thought, man has wondered about his own nature and his place in the world around him. Disputes about the content of the thought of primitive man between, and among, authorities have been frequent and intense.[6] Still, there is little doubt that primitive man has, and has had an image or idea of man which shapes his myths, religions, rituals, mysticism, and folk tales. Abstract conceptions of man, though probably present, are less well substantiated than the images in art, dance, and custom.[7]

In Western European civilization, the earliest, more formally developed theories of man were derived from the Hebrew and Christian Bibles, the Orphic religions, and of course, the organized thought of Plato and Aristotle.[8] Theories of man have abounded ever since from the humanistic orientation of the Renaissance, through the more skeptical Enlightenment, to the existentialists and phenomenologists of more recent times.[9]

St. Augustine, in his spiritual autobiography *The Confessions*, lamented his inability to comprehend his spiritual identity: "I have become a puzzle to myself and this is my infirmity."[10] The anthropological question appears in its plainest form in the Psalms. For example, "What is man, that you should be mindful of him?" (Psalm 8:5) and "Lord what is man that you notice him" (Psalm 144:3).[11] In different ways, the same question recurs in the writing of Camus, Sartre, Heidegger, and in the many tragic heroes and heroines of modern fiction. It underlies the dehumanized painting, music, and architecture of our contemporaries.[12] We still suffer from Augustine's "infirmity." As Rahner puts it, "Man is the question to which there is no answer."[13]

Man's interest in himself as both subject and object of thought should not be surprising. If there is to be a moral life, its aim must be to do good and to avoid evil—but to do good for another human, or to define the nature of the good for humans, that is, we must know the nature of ourselves, others, and the world, otherwise there is no template against which to measure the moral status of our thought and action. The persistence of the anthropological question is a reminder of both our continuing puzzlement and our need to base our moral lives on some concept of the good for humans, that which advances our humanity.

In its most general sense, an anthropology is any formal, systematic, and critical study of the question—What is man? It is in this sense a theory of man. This theory can be organized from a variety of perspectives and methodologies. Depending on which methodology or perspective is employed, anthropologies can be further categorized as physical, social, cultural, philosophical, or theological. Each defines some essential aspect of being human, but none by itself defines the totality of what it is to be a human being. Each is limited by the methodology of the more basic discipline from which it draws its method, that is, natural science, philosophy, theology, the humanities, or the social sciences.

For the purposes of this discussion, I divide anthropologies into theocentric and anthropocentric. The anthropocentric anthropologies may further be classified as scientific, philosophical, or subjectivist in the broad sense common to the literature, history, psychology, and social sciences. The relevant difference for bioethics is the source of moral authority on which ethical decisions are ultimately based. Anthropocentric theories are man-centered. They recognize no ultimate sources of authority beyond man—either as an individual or as a social entity. The theocentric/transcendental theories recognize an ultimate source of moral authority beyond man, that is, in God, some other being, phenomenon of nature, or other "cosmic" force, which imposes moral norms on man.

The distinction I am making can be seen as a continuum: at one end we might place Protagoras and his dictum "Man is the measure of all things."[14] At the other, there is the Catholic Christian dictum that God is the measure of all things, and man is made in God's image and his good is expressed in divine law.[15] Interestingly, the elements of this viewpoint were anticipated in Plato:[16] "Now it is God who is, for you and me, of a truth the measure of all things much more truly than as they say man." Along this continuum, a multitude of "anthropologies" are located, each relating to moral authority in different ways.

Common to all moral discourse is the moment of ethical truth when we must answer the inevitable question of justification. Depending on the theory of man we espouse, we may appeal to sacred scripture, church teachings, the data of empirical science, the correctness of our own reason, moral sentiment, Freudian psychology, common morality, and so on. Ultimately, we end up with free assertions or acts of intellectual or religious faith, because all lines of argument begin with some axiom. When free assertion matches assertion about right and wrong, agreement is no longer possible. This is when, as Plato says, "we become enemies."[17] At this point, the idea of man, the answer we give to the question "What is man?" becomes decisive.

Our theory of man is indeed the Archimedean point of moral discourse. In America at least, the anthropological question is either taken for granted, rejected as meaningless, or declared "off limits." To question another person's ultimate source of moral authority touches on the deepest emotions and identity of the person. To take a deprecating view of another person's ultimate source of moral authority is taken as an attack on that person himself, especially if we speak of "values" instead of moral principles or norms. Talk of "values," because of its subjectivity and relativism does in fact obscure the distinction between persons and their ideas.

Yet, if there is ever to be a better relationship between opposing ethical positions, the anthropological question must be addressed in sustained dialogue. It makes no sense to brand such a dialogue as meaningless. The question will not go away. It hovers over every ethical decision that goes beyond the following of mere procedure. The anthropological question is a foundational and, therefore, a metaphysical question. Foundations and metaphysics are two anathemas for contemporary philosophy, but nonetheless inescapable. Behind every theory of man there is a metaphysics, overt or covert, conscious or unconscious. My focus in this conclusion is on the anthropocentric, man-centered, nontranscendental, and nontheological anthropologies. But in order to set these theories of man in the context of bioethical discourse today, it is useful first to outline one theological, truly transcendental, anthropology and the kind of bioethical system it generates. The Roman Catholic perspective on man is a useful example

because in public debate it is so frequently quoted by those who hold diametrically opposed theories of man and often use it as a foil for man-centered
theories.

One Theocentric Theory: Man as a Spiritual Being

All transcendentally oriented anthropologies define man and the moral
milieu in which he lives in terms of some being or "force" beyond man
himself. This being may be a personal God, as with the Jews, Muslims,
and Christians, or some indefinable but real power in the universe, as with
pantheists or agnostics, or some deity who created the world but does not
intervene in its workings, as with Deists. Transcendental anthropologies
include the traditional "mainline" religions, western and eastern, as well as
modernized forms of the Manichaeism, Gnosticism, and Paganism, often
latent in many forms of "New Age" spirituality. In these cases, moral right
and wrong derive their authority from a source beyond, and superior to,
man, either by direct command, by inference from texts, or from the interpretations of messages and signs of various kinds.

The extent to which these transcendental worldviews influence contemporary bioethics is problematic because the thrust of academic bioethics
in America, at least, is predominantly secular. Roman Catholic theology
is somewhat exceptional in this regard because it has a long history that
predates modern bioethics, going back as a formal study to at least the
fifteenth century.[18] It is also the most quoted counterposition to the secular
anthropocentric anthropologies now dominant in academic settings. This
is especially apparent in the human life questions—end-of-life decisions,
abortion, euthanasia, embryonic stem cell research, cloning, and biotechnological enhancement of human function.

Roman Catholic theology, like Orthodox Jewry, is a paradigm for an
ethic based on an idea of man created by God, to whom God has given life
and a unique nature, and from whom God demands obedience to certain
specific laws. The complexity and breadth of this tradition has been set
forth clearly and in detail in a recent document by the International Theological Commission, an advisory body to the Congregation of the Doctrine
of the Faith.[19] The encyclicals of Pope John Paul II provide a more detailed
philosophical-theological account. *Evangelium vitae*, *Veritatis splendor*,
and *Fides et ratio* are of particular relevance in John Paul II's personalist
idea of man expressed in both his philosophy and theology.[20]

On the Roman Catholic view, human existence is interpreted in accord with the doctrine of *imago dei*, that is, man made in the image of God (Genesis 1:27). This God-given dignity is inherent in every human. It cannot be taken away; it is possessed by all men and women regardless of age, sex, station in life, health or disease, and so forth. In biblical scripture it is expressed in God's covenant with man and his assignment to man of stewardship over the Earth. In a man-centered anthropology, on the other hand, dignity is a socially constructed attribute conferred by individuals on themselves or by others. It is defined on the basis of certain attributes of personhood that can be lost with illness, mental deficiency, disability, state of consciousness, and so on. The sharpest example of dissonance on this point is in the attribution of personal dignity to the embryo from its inception by Catholics, and its categorical denial by others. Some grant "respect" for the embryo but not as a person. Paradoxically, they hold that the embryo can be sacrificed for the good of others to obtain its stem cells for research. Another example is to equate "death" of the person with brain death or with the permanent vegetative state. The very word *vegetative* signifies a loss of dignity incompatible with Roman Catholic moral theology. In the Roman Catholic view, death occurs when all respiratory and cardiovascular functions cease. The Catholic tradition in medical morals antedates modern bioethics by five hundred years.[21] It regards human life as a gift from God, a gift that man must respect and care for.

Anthropocentric Theories of Man

In contrast to theocentric responses to the anthropological question, there are a variety of anthropocentric anthropologies that disavow any possibility or need for a source beyond man himself. Relying solely on man's own reason, emotion, sentiments, and powers of experiment and empirical observation, these man-centered worldviews affirm what is right and good. The "oughtness" or moral compulsions of the moral life stem entirely from man's own will, reflections, and conceptions of his own nature. Man is responsible to himself alone; he is the ultimate measure of all things in the Protagorean sense. He created his own image and idea of himself. He is his own redeemer.

The anthropocentric answers to the anthropological question fall into three major categories, depending on which of man's ways of knowing reality is given primacy of emphasis. One is the *positivist-empirical*, which bases its image and idea of man on that which is observable and testable by the methods of natural science—its object is *man the machine;* second is the *philosophical,* which depends on the ability of human reason to grasp the reality of the moral life and to deduce the good for man from the kind of creature he is—its object is *man the thinker;* the third puts its emphasis on subjectivity, that is, some combination of sentiment, feelings, preferences, intuitive insights, life stories, or emotional experience—its object is man as a *the feeling being.* The method of reflection here is psychological and behavioristic.

The difference between these three broad categories in answer to the question of man lies in the extrapolation of the premises of each, and the way it specifies moral decisions. Each provides a different perception of right and wrong, good and bad human conduct. In the moment of moral decisions, moral agents must act on one idea of man. This "trump" is the ultimate source of a person, or theory's, moral authority and justification. It is the source most resistant to contradiction in the moment of severest challenge. At the moment of decision, one concept or the other will be chosen as the adamantine prelogical basis for all of a person's ultimate ethical justification.

Man as a Machine: The Positivist-Empirical Concept of Man

This approach leans heavily on the findings of biology, physics, and chemistry. For most in academia, the media, and secular bioethics, the positivist-empirical is the preferred idea of man. It represents continuing development of the Cartesian idea of man as a machine, as proposed by Descartes' disciple, la Mettrie.[22] Its major premise is that all of man's body, constitution, and behavior can be explained in terms of chemistry and physics, from physiology to the emotional life and thought itself. In this view, evolution, natural selection, and genetics interact to produce the complexity of human life. But that complexity is the complexity of chemistry and physics.[23]

This point of view has been given tremendous impetus and credibility by the prodigious advances of genetic biology and chemistry. Its adherents admit that there is more to be learned, but they are confident that sooner rather than later we will be able to explain all life, and perhaps even to create it, by the knowledge and techniques of experimental science. Even evolution and natural selection will no longer be chance events, but man-controlled programs for the development of future generations.

In bioethics constructed on this view, man is free to use biotechnology as it deems fit, without restraint, except those that are self-imposed. There is no permanent essence or "nature" of man except his bodily nature evolving according to genetic and evolutionary determinants. Man's body is modifiable for current and future generations with limits set only by man's own determination of desired outcomes. The only "ethical" questions are "Are the outcomes desirable or not?" "Do they produce better or lesser attractive states of affairs?" "Do they produce palpable harm?" Man is the judge of what future generations should be, and should look like. Distinctions between therapy and enhancement are meaningless and naïve. On the positivist view, biotechnology becomes a salvation theme that empowers man to be his own redeemer; Prometheus has been freed by science and is now free to redo the world according to his own plan.

This is the crude form of the scientific-positivist approach. A more sophisticated and gentler variety is offered by the sociobiologist Edward O. Wilson. Wilson is not yet willing to give up some of the aesthetic and social benefits he sees in religion, the arts, and the social sciences. He is willing to sustain them until the day when, he assures us, there will be a true "Consilience"— "an interlocking of causal relationships across disciplines."[24] Wilson believes that "ethics is everything."[25] Once we have arrived at a better understanding of what man is, we will be able to attend better to ethics and prevent losing our humanity. Wilson places his belief in the power of empiricism, but he ends his book wondering if that is really all there is.[26]

More frequently today the anthropological foundation for biomedical ethics is the cruder positivist-empirical view of the Nobelists Watson and Crick. Extrapolations of science's materialist premises produce a bioethics measured by the good of the body or the species, for that is all there is. Mind, soul, emotion, spirit—all are simply epiphenomena of matter, explicable in terms of physics and chemistry. In this view, the old, the sick, the worried, or the disabled are worn-out machines. Some are repairable, some are not. There is no reality beyond what we can touch, see, feel, or smell. Suffering is pointless. When the machinery of the body is irreversibly damaged, death can, and should be, chosen. Euthanasia and assisted suicide, especially the relief of suffering of the elderly and infants, are logical and even desirable. Some would say they are morally mandatory.[27]

In the materialist view, differences between man and other animals are a result of differences in degree of complexity of their brains. The primacy of man in the cosmos rests on this complexity, not on any special moral claim or intrinsic worth. Man is simply one element among the multitude of living things in the biosphere. Some ecologically minded ethicists would give primacy of moral claim to the biosphere, not man. To grant man any primacy would be to be guilty of speciesism—a mortal sin for evolutionary biology.

These are some of the conclusions that follow from the premises of the scientific-empirical anthropological perspective espoused by many bioethicists today. In its extreme form, it converts legitimate science into the ideology of scientism. If we reject the bioethics of a scientistic anthropology, we must look elsewhere for premises that lead to morally more defensible conclusions. This does not mean that the experimental insights and discoveries of the new biology are to be abandoned or denigrated. Good bioethics rests on good science. But science is not ethics. It is invaluable in telling us what man is physically—it is not able to tell us how he should live morally.

Man as a Thinking Being: The Philosophical Concept of Man

Philosophy is the oldest mode of thinking about man and his nature. Man himself and the cosmos were the first subjects on which the earliest Greek philosophers turned their powers of observation and critical reflection. There are evidences that, even for primitive man, man reflected critically on his nature. He examined the knowledge of his senses, but his capacity for reason told him this was not enough.[28]

The philosophy, and particularly the ethics, of Plato, Aristotle, and the Stoics have grounded the most influential conceptions of man in Western ethics, politics, and law. Ancient philosophical inquiry was centered most directly on the question "What is man?" It was the kind of question Socrates, for example, so often asked his friends. As Plato testifies, Socrates was in pursuit of the essence, or *eidos*, of man, the concept that would tell him what makes a thing what it is, and not some other thing. Socrates' dialogue with Euthyphro is illustrative. Socrates asks Euthyphro what holiness is. Socrates wanted to know "the essential aspect by which all holy acts are holy."[29] Euthyphro responds by citing examples of holy persons and holy actions. Socrates repeatedly showed that multiplying examples and details can never add up to an idea, that is, an intellectual representation of the essence of a thing.

Socrates, Plato, and Aristotle arrived at a concept or idea of man by prescinding from the concrete details to arrive at the essence, that aspect by which humans are human. They "peeled" away the accidents, the nonessentials such as age, gender, race, skin color, health, disease, and so forth, the myriad of concrete details that differentiate individuals. What they sought was the irreducible common concept that applied to all those whom we call "man," but not to any other species. They were well aware of the importance of concrete details in other contexts, but not in defining the idea of man, that is, the most general concept applicable to man qua man.

That concept was contained in the notion of man as the being who is rational, animal, and social simultaneously in ways that no other beings can be. It would require a précis of the history of philosophy to show how this idea of man evolved, matured, and became the foundation stone for so much of Western morality. Aristotle, following Plato's inquiry, showed that the function peculiar to man could not be the fact that he is alive, sentient, or animal, but the fact that he can reason and his good is the actualization of this activity.[30] "The good of man is the active exercise of the soul's function in conformity with excellence or virtue."[31]

Aristotle demonstrated the unity of man's material body and his soul. It is the unification and integration of these two elements that constitutes the essence of what it is to be human. The material elements of man are, in this view, susceptible to assessment by the methods of empirical science, and reducible to molecular biology. However, the soul of man, his spiritual essence, cannot be so reduced. The Aristotelian concept of the philosophical unity of body and soul has been recently reviewed in modern terms.[32]

The good for man, in the classical view, is deducible from the idea of man. It cannot be just the good of his body, which is not the whole of man's essence, but of both his body and soul. In this view, man's rationality equips him for reasoned reflection on his own essence and the essences of other beings within the range of his sentient experience. This is not the place to defend the hylomorphism of Aristotle and Aquinas or their successors against the critiques of Locke, Boyle, and others in the seventeenth century. In a less spiritual form, the unity perceived by the Stoics and Cicero survived long enough to become the foundation for the political constructs of the Founding Fathers of the American state.[33]

This idea of man as a rational being, consciously choosing to act and being responsible for his acts, survived as the philosophical basis for ethics more or less intact until Descartes conceptually divided body from soul. From then on, as Gilson points out, the philosophical idea of man lost its unity and thinkers veered toward a host of different theories of man, and consequently of ethics.[34]

Much of modern philosophy repudiates reliance on the classical medieval concept. But, as MacIntyre has shown, remnants of the concept persist in incomplete form in much of contemporary ethics.[35] We can find them in the competing norms of principlism, utilitarianism, deontology, casuistry, social construction, reflective equilibrium, emotivism, and so on. These theories fall within our definition of man-centered, anthropocentric ideas of man and ethics generated by philosophical reflection. Each uses bits and pieces of the classical idea, but not the whole of it. Each does so without the metaphysical grounding that so clearly defined the classical-medieval idea of man. For postmodernists, the deterioration of metaphysics is applauded as freeing bioethics from dogma and cant. For others, it is the major infirmity of contemporary philosophy and bioethics.

Contemporary theories of ethics suffer from the current loss of faith in reason and religion. As a result, many tend to skepticism about moral truths, the possibility of universal norms, and the validity of reason itself. Others see philosophy only as the handmaiden of science, which for all intents and purposes means acceptance of the empiricist-positivist view of man as the basis for a theory of man and bioethics. This subservience of philosophy to science is a crucial consequence of the extradition of metaphysics from both ethics and moral philosophy.

For these reasons, bioethics in the twenty-first century tends to rely on the relativistic, pragmatic, and utilitarian criteria of moral truth.[36] Moral authority is often vested in the philosophy of political liberalism, with its emphasis on personal preference, the invalidity of universal norms of any kind, and the conflation of law and ethics. Bioethical instrumentalism also has wide appeal because it promises the kind of control we would like to have over nature. It breeds the technological hubris so necessary to sustain the ideology of perpetual progress. In the end, one is prompted to ask, how much genuine ethics is left in contemporary bioethics?

Another result of the trends toward an empiricist and a postmodernist concept of man is that many have turned their attention and allegiance away from both science and philosophy. For them, the resources of the humanities and the social sciences seem more promising, more intuitively appealing, and more in touch with the actualities of human experiences of the moral life.

Man as a Feeling Being: The Subjective, Intuitive, Psychodynamic Approach

From the 1970s to the present, there has been a rising tide of disaffection among "humanists" with both the scientific and the philosophical answers to the anthropological question. Many perceive them to be too abstract, rationalistic, and distant from the existential dimensions of what it is to be human and face moral dilemmas. The study of ethics as a discipline is criticized as too formalistic and too formulaic to deal with the richer phenomena of being human.

As an antidote, many now turn for help to literature, the social sciences, or psychology and the behavioral sciences. Their emphasis is on man's affect, consciousness, intuitions, and feelings rather than his rationality. This view has strong affiliations with moral sentiment theories like those of Hutcheson and Hume.[37] Man's existential and not his essential being is, in this view, of primary importance. Emphasis is not on the idea of man—the abstract intellectual representation of his essence—but on his image, that is, his concrete particularized uniqueness as perceived in an individual. In classical terms, images are defined in terms of "accidentals"—those concrete attributes that identify individuals as particular persons. An image speaks to the being of *this* person; an idea speaks to what all persons *are*. An image is an example of an entity, not an expression of what makes an entity what it is. Images are important to any full understanding of what it is to be human. Images help us to comprehend the moral dilemma of a particular person. But images of a particular person's moral life cannot be extrapolated as a norm for all human life. As descriptive entities, they are invaluable, as concepts, they are not.

Philosophy, classically at least, has prescinded from precisely those things that particularize a concrete entity. Ethics seeks a norm that can guide us to good behavior for all man—not just a particular man. Today's psychology, behavioral sciences, and sociology describe what a person looks like, how he behaves, what he feels, how he relates to others and to society, that is, what makes each person a unique being. There is no question that these individualizing components are crucial to understanding the moral life. They are essential to a complete understanding of the experience of being, that is, of being a human being.

When making a judgment about the morality of a particular human being's particular acts, moral psychology must be taken into consideration. However, these particulars by themselves do not suffice to give moral justification to an act. Remembering Euthyphro, we cannot leap from a multiplication of examples or details of the moral psychology of a moral agent to the rectitude of his moral decisions or acts. We need a template beyond, that is, an idea of man and the good against which to measure or prescribe right and wrong. Lacking this template we are left with competing stories and no way to judge their moral probity.

Facts about the psychological, social, and emotional milieu of a moral act help us to understand why and how a person acts in a particular difficult moral situation. But to make a moral judgment we must have an idea of man, a conception of the good for humans that transcends the good perceived by an individual person for himself.

The moral psychology of a moral act is often decisive in assessing culpability and degrees of guilt. Notions of moral culpability have always depended on the concrete setting, the personal and interpersonal relationships of a moral decision or act. The delineation of characters is the material out of which great writers, mystics, and today's psychologists lead us to a sympathetic and empathetic grasp of another person's moral dilemmas. Well-drawn characters arouse a cofeeling for the anguish and difficulty of moral choice and a desire to help in some way. The extenuating circumstances of individual acts cannot, however, alter the fact that certain acts are morally wrong in themselves.

The feelings evoked by a creative writer do not tell us if our judgment based on these feelings is right or wrong. Characters such as Antigone, Ulysses, Hamlet, Meursault, or the thousands of others from world literature may invoke our sympathy or our disgust. We must still decide, however, if their acts and intentions are morally justified. If we judge characters in literature or fiction as paragons of either vice or virtue, how do we justify our ethical appraisal?

Bioethics based on an affective or intuitive answer to the anthropological question too easily psychologizes ethics. Ethics turns from norms to questions of "values" without the benefit of an axiology to ground those values beyond personal preference. Moral judgments then are justified if they "feel" good or make one "comfortable."

The intuitive approach to ethics based in images rather than ideas is powerfully reinforced by the ubiquitous electronic barrage of image to which we are constantly exposed. The medium is indeed the message. We no longer look to books or thought for truth, but in electronic images. For many, these are their major, or only, instruments for contact with reality. Argumentation about morals becomes not so much a search for understanding, but an expression of feelings to which we are entitled simply because they are our own.

Stories have a long and honorable history in the teaching of morals. Indeed, stories are the oldest devices for bringing immediacy and concreteness to moral discourse. We can think of Hebrew and Christian Bibles, the Greek drama, the fables of Aesop, and the multitude of characters created by the great writers of every epoch. From Antigone to Hamlet to the tragic heroes and heroines of modern literature, great writers draw us into the concrete realities of moral choice.

All true literature, intentionally or not, poses moral questions.[38] The author works with an imagined laboratory in which the dilemmas of being human are played out in a thousand creative ways. The concreteness of a fictional character's life experiences evokes vicarious experiences in the reader. The writer's skills can pull us into the story. We cannot avoid some identification with the character's moral dilemmas, and we cannot help judging and examining our own lives in ways an abstract discussion cannot match.

Despite Sophocles' powerful portrayal of Antigone's resistance to Creon, we must ask, "Was she a brave and virtuous heroine who defied the law to honor the custom of burial of the dead? Was she a dangerous rebel, threatening the order of the Theban state? Or was she, as Jean Anouilh portrays her, an immature neurotic adolescent?"[39] After Sophocles, a multitude of others have retold the story of Antigone, each with a different view of her character. As Steiner has said, Antigone is the paradigm case for moral issues of the greatest moment.[40]

Stories have universal appeal, but our judgments of their moral lessons must go beyond aesthetic appeal. Only if we accept the author as morally authoritative, and beyond question, can a story have moral authority. Even when the author is God, competing exegeses of biblical texts show how difficult it is to translate even authoritative sources into agreed-upon moral action guidelines.

Is Productive Dialogue between Competing Anthropologies Possible?

Given the disparities in the types of theories of man I have suggested, what are the possibilities of productive dialogue between, and among, them? Each theory calls on a different source of moral authority to justify its norms. Some of them look to transcendent sources, some to man himself. Each theory, when extrapolated to its logical conclusion, yields a different system of bioethics. Yet, if we are as humans to confront the challenges and dilemmas of contemporary biotechnology, there must be some source of common agreement on what is, and what is not, morally congruent with what it means to be human.

The difficulties of engagement between the disparate theories of man are obvious. They have resulted in polarized positions on virtually every one of the most important ethics issues affecting humankind. Yet it is of the nature of these issues to transcend national, geographical, cultural, and political boundaries. The human life questions affect all of us simply because they are questions common to our shared humanity. They cannot be confined within fragmented communities of value, ignorant of and hostile to each other. Not only are we moral strangers, but we are in danger of becoming moral enemies as well.

Given these difficulties, where should the requisite dialogue begin? What are the minimum conditions for initiating a dialogue that will respect differences while seeking what is common to our shared humanity?

A first step, surely, is the admission that every anthropology—that is, every theory of man—grasps some essential aspect of man's existence. The difference in each theory is its contribution to our better understanding of the whole. A full grasp of our humanity is inconceivable, however, without some accord on what we can agree is common to our shared humanity, and therefore what must be safeguarded in our moral norms and values.

Finding this common ground does not mean capitulation of all to one or the other of the competing theories I have discussed. Nor must it suggest that opposing views on certain postulates are irreconcilable (abortion, euthanasia) and cannot be subject to negotiation or compromise. Neither does it mean sacrifice of our deepest convictions about the ultimate sources of morality simply to gain consensus. Somehow we must distinguish between those moral decisions that are universally binding and those that can best be held in private. Where those lines are drawn will be the source of much debate without easy resolution.

The sharpest divide will continue to be between the theocentric and the anthropocentric theories of man. If dialogue is to have any possibility here, it will require openness—not capitulation—especially between religion and science and the different ways of their knowing. Einstein, who did not believe in a personal God, and had serious doubts about institutionalized religion, nonetheless saw clearly where the disjunction and conjunction could be located: "Scientific method can teach us nothing else beyond how facts are related to, and are conditioned by, each other . . . yet it is equally clear that knowledge of what *is* does not open the door directly to what *should be*."[41]

Einstein's sage observation requires some restraint on the hubris of both science and religion. Those who build their idea of man on faith and revelation must acknowledge the validity of the scientific method for those aspects of man susceptible to that method. If they are to be critical of science, it must be in recognizing that all science is at the core a search for a god who created this awesome universe. To be valid, a critique of science by believers must be based in good science if the data and conclusions of science as science are at issue.

Correspondingly, those who contribute to our fund of empirical and experimental knowledge must rein in their hubris when the issue transcends the method of science. To tell us all how to live and resolve the ethical dilemmas resulting from our increased powers over nature, the scientists must be willing to recognize the limitations of science in moral matters. If scientists are to criticize moral norms, they must be willing to engage them on terms suitable to the discourse. The current tendency to scientific triumphalism on the part of those who have made important scientific discoveries is damaging to genuine dialogue, as is religious triumphalism.

To affect this kind of mutual respect, some score of "gray zone" people need to be trained in our universities. By this, I mean some practicing scientists must study philosophy and ethics seriously and be competent enough to speak and write knowledgeably in both fields. The same must be said of theologians, some of whom must be well-schooled in one of the relevant sciences. These "bridge" intellects can do much to close the gap between science and religion in accordance with Einstein's concise delineation of their respective roles in human affairs. It is difficult but necessary for a small cadre of "gray zone" scholars to cultivate the territory between science and religion.

Given these disparities, what possibility is there for a satisfactory response to the plea of the president's council for help in deciding which technologies enhance, and which diminish, our humanity? The council itself turned to one source—the world's literature—to draw inspiration from the evocative power of the world's great writers, ancient and modern. As suggested earlier, this is a direction that will enrich our understandings of man's existential experiences. It is not of itself sufficient. It needs to be complimented by consideration of the *idea* as well as by the *image* of man.

The difficulties of such an engagement are obvious, especially now, because opposing ideas and images have become so polarized. Nonetheless, before we decide that opposing positions are irreconcilable, the effort must be made to maintain the dialogue between them. The consequences of not doing so are socially too consequential to be ignored.

To this end, one may turn, at a minimum, to the conditions under which dialogue and dialect might be fruitfully pursued.

We can begin with the fact that every theory of man grasps some essential aspect of man's nature, and this is its contribution to the whole. This openness of each view to the value of the other applies to the emphasis on images in the psychosocial and literary theories of man as well as the more abstract conceptual perspectives. A full grasp of what man is becomes impossible without recognizing some synthesis of image and idea, of concrete existence and abstract essence.

The convictions of academic bioethics and materialist conceptions of man that religion has no place in bioethical discourse needs reassessment. There is little likelihood of agreement with any general set of ethical norms if we fail to recognize that the majority of the world's peoples have some kind of commitment to belief in the spiritual and transcendental. Blaise Pascal, no mean scientist himself, put it this way: "God alone can teach us the knowledge of our nature which of ourselves we cannot have."[42]

This does not mean conversion or a faith commitment for atheists or agnostics. It does mean a readiness to take into account the almost universal yearning for the spiritual in the lives of most humans. It does mean that religion cannot justly be disenfranchised as it is so often in today's academic secular bioethical discourse.

Speaking of conversion, productive dialogue does not mean the eclipse of all other theories by one theory. Materialists are convinced that chemistry and physics have given us the key to everything it means to be human.[43] Edward O. Wilson is more tolerant for the moment of the contributions of the social sciences, the humanities, and religion. He believes in the end, however, that all disciplines will be reducible to empiricism fused in the crucible of Consilience.[44]

While fully appreciating the difficulties, there is growing evidence of the dialogue between the positivist-empirical and the theological ideas of man built on some of the conditions outlined earlier. Substantial differences persist, of course, but the disastrous practical consequences of a widening gulf of understanding and action are sufficiently apparent to impel better communication. These examples are the published reports of the president's council on bioethics (1–5); the UN Universal Declaration on Human Rights (1948), and the current drafts of the UNESCO International Committee on Bioethics on the subject of universal norms on bioethics. This is not the place to review the content of these publications. They do demonstrate, however, that there are substantial areas of agreement (as well as disagreement), but that dialogue and consensus statements are achievable.

The UN Declaration on Human Rights is just slightly more than fifty years old (1948). One finds here a clear statement of the inherent dignity and equality of all members of the human family. This assertion is made clearly in the preamble and developed in thirty subsequent articles. One may quarrel with wording, inclusion, or exclusion of some item or other. The emphasis of the articles is more legal than moral. But all the "rights" are grounded in the opening principle of the dignity inherent in the human person—an idea of man that is essentially a being distinctly worthy of respect.

A second example is the ongoing current dialogue in the draft document of UNESCO's International Committee on Bioethics titled "Preliminary Draft Declaration on Universal Norms of Bioethics." At this writing, this document is working its way through the UNESCO approval process, and its final form is not yet fixed (February 9, 2005, draft). What is notable again is the measure of agreement on important ethical norms among representatives of many nations, cultures, and religious traditions.

This document, like the UN declaration, begins with the following statement: "Any decision or practice shall be made or carried out with full respect for the inherent dignity of the human person, human rights and fundamental freedoms. Any decision or practice shall respect the principle that the interests and welfare of the human person prevail over the interest of science or society."[45] Some thirty articles follow, based on these principles, including respect for cultural diversity, job discrimination, autonomy, informed consent, privacy and confidentiality, solidarity, social responsibility, and stewardship for the biosphere, as well as the principles for implementation of these principles.

As with the UN declaration and the reports of the president's council, one may quarrel with certain emphases, inclusion or exclusion of certain principles, wording, and so forth. Those of us who hold to a theocentric anthropology find no explicit recognition of a personal God. The tendency to legalistic rather than moral phraseology is troublesome. Likewise, the reference to "reproductive rights" (Article 13a, February 9, 2005, draft) would not be acceptable if it implied abortion or certain other reproductive technologies.

However, taken as a whole, the UNESCO declaration modifies a set of bioethical moral norms to which those who hold differing anthropologies can give assent in principle. This measure of agreement is remarkable considering the differences in language, culture, and world perspectives among the members of the drafting committee. This assessment must be tempered by the fact that the declarations of the United Nations, UNESCO, and the president's council can be criticized as "consensus ethics." In the end, negotiation between conflicting ethical positions is not a defensible mechanism for arriving at moral truth.

However, certain moral norms and principles are so self-evident that they can be consistent with widely differing worldviews and anthropologies. This is the case not because we have agreement on the truth of these norms but because these norms are universally and self-evidently true. This reflects in large part a natural law approach, as adumbrated by Aristotle and developed in more detail by Thomas Aquinas.[46]

Natural law ethics so conceived is based solely on reason. It is distinct from theological or scriptural authority. It is open to all persons irrespective of their theological persuasions or the absence thereof. As a result, the natural law ethic binds all reasoning persons, not just believers. Its precepts are, for both believers and nonbelievers, self-evident truths. They cannot be proven; they need no proof. They are necessary predicates to any idea of man as he existed in the past and exists today. They are what defines man ontologically.

Dignity could be classified in terms of modern day analytic philosophy as an analytic a priori postulate, as Gómez-Lobo has suggested.[47] These postulates are thus products of reasoning unassisted by divine revelation or acts of faith, except in the first principles of reasoning itself. They can therefore be bridges for dialogue between competing anthropologies.

Dignity appears as a first principle in documents as diverse as those prepared by the secular declarations of the United Nations on human rights, of UNESCO on norms of bioethics, and also in the Catholic Christian anthropology of the International Theological Commission. For the nonbeliever, man's inherent dignity is a self-evident truth of unaided human reason; for the believer, it is also a self-evident truth open to reason, but immensely enriched by biblical and Church teaching (Genesis 1:27).

The concept of human dignity is one example of the way philosophy, particularly the natural law moral philosophy, can act as the bridge between believers and nonbelievers. Philosophy is, as McInerny says so well, "the *lingua franca*, enabling believers and non-believers to come together in the recognition of naturally known truths."[48] One need not accept the whole of the Aristotelian-Thomist conception of man to sustain the dialogue. Yet such other self-evident truths as human dignity, rationality, and human social and political inclinations can provide bridges over which moral dialogue can proceed.

In *Man and History*, Max Scheler pointed gloomily to the bafflement of modern man with his own identity: "In the ten thousand years of history we are the first age in which man has become utterly and unconditionally problematic to himself, in which he no longer knows who he is, but at the same time knows that he does not know."[49]

In the twenty-first century, we seem certain to know much more about man as a biological being, but probably not much more about who, what, and why he is. But we cannot any longer, especially in bioethics, abandon the anthropological question as "utterly problematic." For better or worse, we have the power to alter our biological makeup in still unimagined ways. Without a clearer idea of what man *is*, we will enter and remain in a dark moral forest without a compass.

NOTES

1. President's Council on Bioethics, *Being Human: Readings from the President's Council on Bioethics* (Washington, DC: U.S. Government Printing Office, 2003), xx.

2. Ernst Cassirer, *An Essay on Man* (New Haven, CT: Yale University Press, 1992), 1.

3. Max Scheler, *Die Stellung des Menschen in Kosmos* (Darmstadt, Ger.: Reichl, 1928), 18f. Cited in Cassirer, *Essay on Man*, 22.

4. Lars Reuter, *Modern Biotechnology in Postmodern Times: A Reflection on European Policies and Human Agency* (Dordrecht, Neth.: Kluwer Academic Publishers, 2003), 3.

5. Roberto Dell'Oro, this volume.

6. Sir James George Fraser, *The New Golden Bough: A New Abridgment of the Classic Work*, ed. Theodor H. Gaster (Great Meadows, NJ: S. G. Phillips, 1959); Lucien Lévy-Bruhl, *The "Soul" of the Primitive* (London: Allen and Unwin, 1965).

7. Paul Radin, *Primitive Man as Philosopher* (New York: D. Appleton and Company, 1927), 275–91.

8. Mieczy[s]law Albert Krapiec, *I-man: An Outline of Philosophical Anthropology*, trans. Marie Lescoe et al. (New Britain, CT: Mariel Publications, 1983), 2–3; Cassirer, *Essay on Man*.

9. Maurice S. Friedman, *To Deny Our Nothingness: Contemporary Images of Man* (New York: Delacorte Press, 1967); Maurice Merleau-Ponty, "Phenomenology and the Sciences of Man," in *Phenomenology and the Social Sciences*, ed. Maurice Natason (Evanston, IL: Northwestern University Press, 1973), 74; Francisco Romero, *Theory of Man*, trans. William F. Cooper (Berkeley: University of California Press, 1964), xxxi; Michael Polanyi, *The Study of Man* (Chicago: Chicago University Press, 1959); Paul Edwards, ed., *The Encyclopedia of Philosophy*, vol. 6 (New York: Macmillan, 1976), 159–60.

10. Saint Augustine, *Confessions: Books I–XIII*, trans. F. J. Sheed (Indianapolis, IN: Hackett, 1993), X:198.

11. Biblical citations refer to *The New American Bible* (New York.: P. J. Kennedy, 1970).

12. José Ortega y Gasset, *The Dehumanization of Art, and Other Writings on Art and Culture* (New York: Doubleday, 1948), 8–13.

13. Karl Rahner, "What Is Man?" in *Christian at the Crossroads* (New York: Seabury Press, 1975), 11.

14. Plato, *Theatetus*, in *The Collected Dialogues of Plato, Including the Letters*, ed. Edith Hamilton and Huntington Cairns, trans. F. M. Cornford (Princeton, NJ: Princeton University Press, 1982), 852, line 152a.

15. The International Theological Commission, "Communion and Stewardship: Human Persons Created in the Image of God," *Origins* 34, no. 15 (2004): 234–48.

16. Plato, *The Laws*, IV, in *The Collected Dialogues of Plato, Including the Letters*, ed. Hamilton and Cairns, 1307, line 716c.

17. Plato, *Euthyphro*, trans. Harold North Fowler (Cambridge, MA: Harvard University Press, 1977), 27.

18. David F. Kelly, *The Emergence of Roman Catholic Medical Ethics in North America: An Historical-Methodological-Bibliographical Study* (New York: Edward Mellon Press, 1979), 98–101.

19. The International Theological Commission, "Communion and Stewardship: Human Persons Created in the Image of God," *Origins* 34, no. 15 (2004): 234–48.

20. Pope John Paul II, "Encyclical Letter: Evangelium Vitae," *Libreria Editrice Vaticana: John Paul II—Encyclicals with Study Tool*, March 25, 1995, available at www.vatican.va/holy_father/john_paul_ii/encyclicals/ (accessed May 24, 2005); Pope John Paul II, "Encyclical Letter: Veritatis Splendor," *Libreria Editrice Vaticana*, August 6, 1993, available at www.vatican.va/holy_father/john_paul_ii/encyclicals/ (accessed May 24, 2005); Pope John Paul II, "Encyclical Letter: Fides et Ratio," *Libreria Editrice Vaticana*, September 14, 1998, available at www.vatican.va/holy_father/john_paul_ii/encyclicals/ (accessed May 24, 2005); Avery Dulles, "John Paul II and the Mystery of the Human Person," *America* 190, no. 3 (2004): 10–21; Kenneth L. Schmitz, *At the Center of the Human Drama: The Philosophical Anthropology of Karol Wojtyla/Pope John Paul II* (Washington, DC: Catholic University of America Press, 1993); Martin Cyril D'Arcy, *Humanism and Christianity* (Cleveland, OH: Meridian Books, 1970).

21. Kelly, *Emergence of Roman Catholic Medical Ethics in North America*, 98–101.

22. Julien Offray de La Mettrie, *L'Homme Machine: A Study in the Origins of an Idea* (Princeton, NJ: Princeton University Press, 1960).

23. James D. Watson with Andrew Berry, *DNA: The Secret of Life* (New York: Alfred A. Knopf, 2003).

24. Edward O. Wilson, *Consilience: The Unity of Knowledge* (New York: Knopf, 1998), 235.

25. Ibid., 297.

26. Ibid., 297–98.

27. Jan Hendrik van den Berg, *Medical Power and Medical Ethics* (New York: W.W. Norton and Company, 1969).

28. Radin, *Primitive Man as Philosopher*.

29. Plato, *Euthyphro*, 23.

30. Giovanni Reale, "Plato and Aristotle," in *A History of Ancient Philosophy*, vol. 2, trans. John R. Catan (New York: SUNY Press, 1987), 319–20.

31. Aristotle, *The Complete Works of Aristotle: The Revised Oxford Translation*, vol. 2, ed. Jonathan Barnes (Princeton, NJ: Princeton University Press, 1984), NE 1097b 22–1098a 20.

32. Jason T. Eberl, "Aquinas on the Nature of Human Beings," *The Review of Metaphysics* 58, no. 2 (2004): 164.

33. Morton White, *The Philosophy of the American Revolution* (New York: Oxford University Press, 1981); Carl J. Richard, *The Founders and the Classics: Greece, Rome, and the American Enlightenment* (Cambridge, MA: Harvard University Press, 1994).

34. Etienne Gilson, *The Unity of Philosophical Experience* (New York: C. Scribner's Sons, 1937), 173–75.

35. Alasdair MacIntyre, *After Virtue: A Study in Moral Theory* (Notre Dame, IN: University of Notre Dame Press, 1981).

36. Edmund D. Pellegrino, "Bioethics at Century's Turn: Can Normative Ethics Be Retrieved?" *Journal of Medicine and Philosophy* 25 (2000): 655–75.

37. Francis Hutcheson, *An Essay on the Nature and Conduct of the Passions and Affections* (1728; repr., Menston, England: Scolar Press, 1972); David Hume, *A Treatise on Human Nature*, ed. L. A. Selby-Bigge and P. H. Nidditch (1737; repr., Oxford: Clarendon Press, 1975).

38. John Gardner, *On Moral Fiction* (New York: Basic Books, 1978).

39. Jean Anouilh, *Antigone*, trans. Barbara Bray (1944; repr., London: Methuen, 2000).

40. George Steiner, *Antigones* (New York: Oxford University Press, 1984).

41. Albert Einstein, *Out of My Later Years* (Secaucus, NJ: Citadel, 1956), 21–22.

42. Blaise Pascal, *Pensées*, trans. H. F. Stewart (New York: Pantheon Books, 1950), 141.

43. Watson with Berry, *DNA*.

44. Wilson, *Consilience*.

45. UNESCO (United Nations Educational, Scientific and Cultural Organization), 2005, available at www.unesco.org (accessed May 25, 2005).

46. Saint Thomas Aquinas, *Summa Theologiae*, vol. 2, trans. Fathers of the English Dominican Province, Ia, IIae, Article 94 (Allen, TX: Christian Classics, 1948), I–II, Question 94, 1009–10; Alfonso Gómez-Lobo, *Morality and the Human Goods: An Introduction to Natural Law Ethics* (Washington, DC: Georgetown University Press, 2002), 126–28; Germain Gabriel Grisez, "The First Principle of Practical Reason: A Commentary on the *Summa Theologiae* I–II, Question 94, Article 2," *Natural Law Forum* 10 (1965): 168–201.

47. Gómez-Lobo, *Morality and the Human Goods,* 126–28; Saul Kripke, "Identity and Necessity," in *Naming, Necessity and Natural Kinds* (New York: Cornell University Press, 1977), 66–101.

48. Ralph M. McInerny, foreword, *A Short History of Thomism,* by Romanus Cessario (Washington, DC: Catholic University of America Press, 2005), x.

49. Max Scheler, "Man and History," in *Man's Place in Nature,* trans. Hans Myerhoff (New York: Farrar Straus and Cudahy, 1962), xiii.

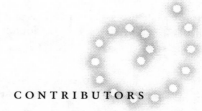

CONTRIBUTORS

Lisa Sowle Cahill is J. Donald Monan Professor, Theology Department, Boston College.

Alisa L. Carse is associate professor, Department of Philosophy, Georgetown University.

Roberto Dell'Oro is assistant professor in The Bioethics Institute and the graduate director of the Master of Arts Program in Bioethics at Loyola Marymount University.

William Desmond is professor of philosophy, Institute of Philosophy, Katholieke Universiteit Leuven, Belgium, and David Cook Visiting Chair in Philosophy at Villanova University.

Kevin T. FitzGerald, S.J., is David Lauler Chair in Catholic Health Care Ethics, Center for Clinical Bioethics, and research associate professor in the Department of Oncology, Georgetown University Medical Center.

Christine E. Gudorf is professor, Department of Religious Studies, Florida International University.

Ron Hamel is senior director, ethics, The Catholic Health Association of the United States.

Suzanne Holland is associate professor of religious and social ethics, and chair of the Department of Religion, University of Puget Sound.

M. Therese Lysaught is associate professor of religious studies, University of Dayton.

Margaret E. Mohrmann is associate professor of religious studies and associate professor of pediatrics and medical education, University of Virginia.

Edmund D. Pellegrino is professor emeritus of medicine and medical ethics, Center for Clinical Bioethics, Georgetown University.

Daniel P. Sulmasy, O.F.M., is Sisters of Charity Chair in Ethics, St. Vincent's Hospital, Manhattan, and professor of medicine and director of The Bioethics Institute, New York Medical College.

Carol Taylor, C.S.F.N., is director, Center for Clinical Bioethics, Georgetown University.

S. Kay Toombs is associate professor emeritus of philosophy, Baylor University.

Richard M. Zaner is Anne Geddes Stahlman Professor Emeritus of Medical Ethics and Philosophy of Medicine, Vanderbilt University Medical Center.

INDEX

Printed in the United States
133251LV00005B/54/A

9 781589 010796